GET ON IT!
BOSU® Balance Trainer

GET ON IT!

BOSU® Balance Trainer

Workouts for Core Strength and a Super-Toned Body

JANE ARONOVITCH, MIRIANE TAYLOR, COLLEEN CRAIG

Photography by **Andy Mogg**

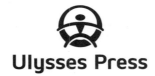

Ulysses Press

Published in the United States by Ulysses Press
P.O. Box 3440
Berkeley, CA 94703
www.ulyssespress.com

ISBN13: 978-1-56975-589-1
Library of Congress Control Number 2007906111

Printed in the United States by Bang Printing

10 9 8 7 6

Editorial/Production	Lily Chou, Claire Chun, Steven Zah Schwartz, Elyce Petker, Lauren Harrison, Abigail Reser, Tamara Kowalski
Index	Sayre Van Young
Cover design	what!design @ whatweb.com
Photography	Andy Mogg
Models	Miriane Taylor, Jane Aronovitch, Herman Chan, Emily Butts

Distributed by Publishers Group West

Please Note
This book has been written and published strictly for informational purposes, and in no way should be used as a substitute for consultation with health care professionals. You should not consider educational material herein to be the practice of medicine or to replace consultation with a physician or other medical practitioner. The author and publisher are providing you with information in this work so that you can have the knowledge and can choose, at your own risk, to act on that knowledge. The author and publisher also urge all readers to be aware of their health status and to consult health care professionals before beginning any health program.

Note to Readers
BOSU® is a registered trademark of BOSU Fitness, LLC and is protected under United States and international laws and is used under license from BOSU Fitness, LLC. The views expressed in this book are not endorsed by BOSU Fitness, LLC, and the author(s) of this book are in no way affiliated with, or sponsored by BOSU Fitness, LLC.

part 1:
getting
started

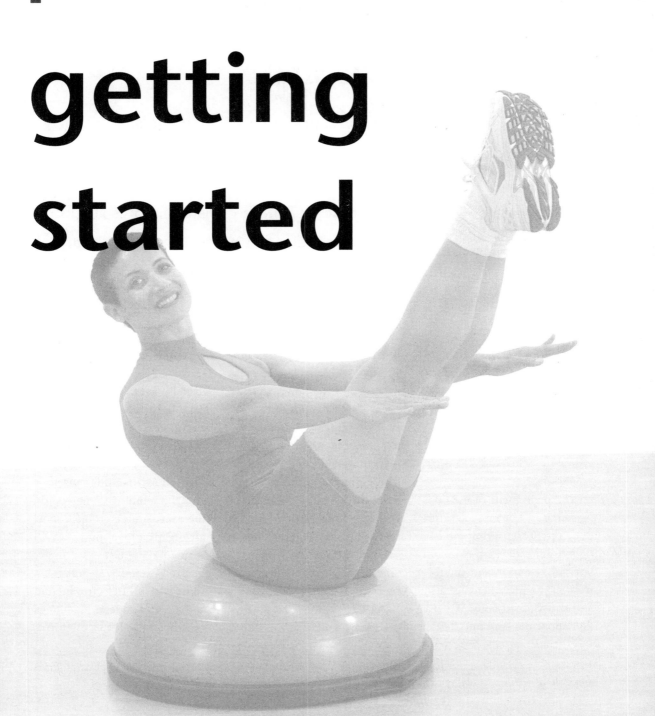

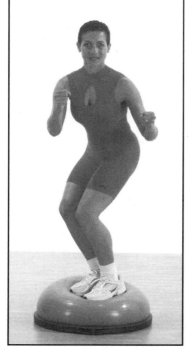

about the book

Welcome to *Get on It! BOSU Balance Trainer: Workouts for Core Strength and a Super-Toned Body*. With all the buzz about core training and more and more gyms and stores stocking BOSUs, we decided it was time to write a book about the BOSU and how to use it to develop a strong core and toned body.

Get on It! BOSU Balance Trainer is primarily a "how-to" book for anyone who wants to work with a BOSU, whether you have little or no experience or are an experienced enthusiast who wants to hone your skills.*

The main focus of the book is exercises, but first we introduce the BOSU and discuss how it helps develop core strength, balance, and stability—all the ingredients of a fit and super-toned body. We also talk about the core muscles:

what they are, where they're located, and what they do.

Part 2 of the book presents BOSU basics. It offers a series of warm-up exercises and explains how to stand and start to move on the dome. The examples in this section form the basis for the exercises that appear in Part 3.

Part 3 is devoted to exercises of various types. For simplicity we've grouped them by exercise type—squats and lunges, back exercises, and so on. Please note that the cate-

gories are not absolute. For example, you may find an exercise in the Kneeling section that works the abs really strenuously. That's because, unlike some workout regimens, most of the BOSU exercises work more than one muscle group at a time. In other words, the exercises are grouped more for organizational purposes than anything else.

Each exercise category starts with a brief introduction and a list of general guidelines called Helpful Hints. Within a

---

* *Regardless of your level of experience with the BOSU, we assume that readers have a basic level of physical fitness and skill, as well as the ability to judge how far to go and when to stop.*

category, each exercise shows a starting position and gives step-by-step instructions for each move. We've also incorporated plenty of illustrative photos of the steps. Following each exercise is a list of relevant Tips—ideas to keep in mind or cues to help with execution. We also include some Basic variations if you want to simplify a particular move, as well as Challenge and Super-challenge variations if you're seeking to push yourself a little harder.

Part 4 contains a series of suggested workouts. Some focus on specific muscle groups, while others are complete workouts with a warm-up, full set of exercises, and stretches at the end. You can use these workouts exclusively, move through the book sequentially, or pick and choose moves that particularly interest you. In any case, we hope you enjoy the book and develop the same passion for the BOSU that we have!

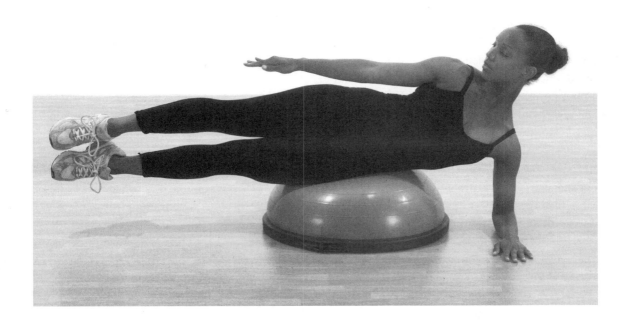

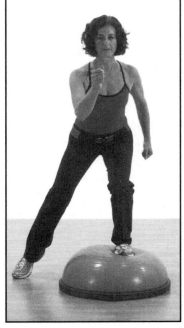

the buzz about BOSU

Short for "both sides utilized," the BOSU Balance Trainer,® or BOSU (pronounced "Bo" like the boy's name, and "Sue" like the girl's name), was invented by Californian David Weck in 1999 and launched in 2000. Since then it has become one of the most popular fitness tools in the industry.

The BOSU is approximately 25 inches wide and looks like a big exercise ball that's been cut in half. One side is dome-shaped; the other is flat. The dome side is inflatable and should be filled with air using a pump until it is fairly firm and about eight to ten inches high.

Through its ingenious construction, the BOSU has two unstable surfaces that transform even the simplest moves into a fun and challenging workout. Working on an uneven surface tests your balance and forces you to use and strengthen deep core and stabilizing muscles—muscles that conventional exercise programs often miss.

Suitable for all ages and fitness levels, the BOSU can be used at home or in studio or gym classes. Trainers, athletes, dancers, and general fitness buffs alike use the BOSU to build strength and agility, tone and sculpt muscles, improve aerobic conditioning, burn fat, and improve posture and alignment.

Looking for that long, lean look? The BOSU can help you trim down your waistline. You can also use the BOSU to combine aerobic and cardiovascular exercises with strength training, balance challenges, and flexibility— all the components of a well-rounded exercise regimen.

Making the right connections

Most trainers and sports practitioners agree that a successful core-strengthening program targets groups of muscles in a coordinated way. Some people refer to this approach as functional or integrative training—training the whole body based on the idea that this is how we move in our daily activities.

In his book *The Athlete's Ball*, Rick Jemmett states: "Integrative training exercises

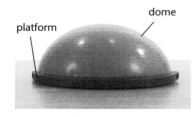

platform

dome

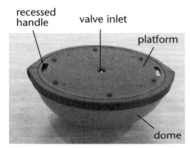

recessed handle

valve inlet

platform

dome

BOSU Balance Trainer

require the spinal joints plus varying combinations of ankle, knee, hip, shoulder, elbow, and wrist joints, and all the muscles which function at these joints, to work together to perform a given exercise." Jemmett, a physical therapist who specializes in lower back pain, uses the BOSU and stability ball to train athletes as well as help people with injuries. He explains that integrative training exercises "require us to support our body weight, stabilize our core, work our arms or legs, and, in some exercises, lift heavy weights, all at the same time" *(Jemmett 2004, p. 7)*.

Even something as simple as standing on the BOSU is an example of working the body in an integrated way. As soon as you step on the dome, you feel all the muscles in your body come alive. That feeling is even stronger as you start to move and change positions. For example, when we lift one leg or one arm, our weight shifts and our body has to quickly adjust to this change. When we expand our repertoire to move the upper and lower torso or to work one side of the body and then the other, we need the simultaneous participation of the entire body and quick and flexible motor control. These are all examples of integrated training.

While Jemmett said the following with reference to a stability ball, the same holds true for the BOSU. It "provides an unstable support surface, which stimulates the body's stabilizing mechanisms. This allows you to train the function of the muscles and not just their strength" *(Jemmett 2004, p. 7)*.

It seems clear that by its very nature the BOSU is designed to help people strengthen their core and exercise in an integrated way. This is, indeed, the power and beauty of the BOSU and, by association, the exercises that appear in this book. We hope you enjoy them and derive the same pleasure and satisfaction from your BOSU workouts as we do.

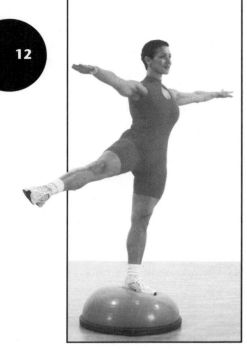

a balancing act

What is balance and why is it so important? In the context of movement, when we talk about balance we usually mean holding a certain body position, perhaps for a period of time. Sounds simple, right? But balancing is actually a very complicated process. There's a lot going on in the body when we try to balance.

Here's what it boils down to. The brain uses feedback from a number of built-in sensing systems in our bodies—our eyes, our ears, our inner ears, our skin, our muscles, and more—to help us figure out where we are in space. The brain then processes and uses that information to transmit signals back to our muscles so we can react accordingly.

Generally, the more we practice balancing, the better we become. In other words, we can train ourselves to balance better.

Improving our balance is desirable because balance is a part of all movement. Even the act of walking—essentially transferring the weight from one foot to the other—involves a moment of balance in between. It therefore follows that improving balance enhances the performance of any movement—in exercise programs, sports, or general activities of daily living.

That's where the BOSU comes in. It targets—and trains—the muscles you need to balance and stabilize, almost without having to think about it. Working with the BOSU not only helps you improve your balance but also helps you develop more control, and execute all your movements with more grace and agility.

Working on an unstable surface

As noted above, our bodies have a built-in mechanism to detect where we are in space. It all depends on the brain's ability to figure out where every part of our body is relative to every other part, and then make appropriate neuromuscular adjustments so we can move or balance effectively.

When you stand on a flat surface, like a solid floor, you send feedback from that floor, through your feet, and up the

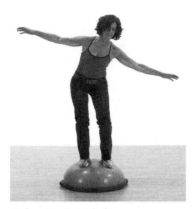

Balancing is tricky!

"kinetic chain" to your brain. However, when you stand on a rounded surface, like the top of a BOSU, you send a very different message, with a lot more, and probably new, information for your brain to process.

For this reason, when you first stand on a BOSU, you may find that you move around quite a bit. Each movement—even each wobble—sends a signal to your brain about how your base of support and center of gravity have changed. This forces the body to make constant adjustments to maintain balance with each movement.

With so much new and different information for the brain to process, or maybe also because the muscles you need to respond appropriately aren't sufficiently trained yet, you may find yourself wobbling quite a bit as your body tries to make sense of where you are, especially at the beginning of your BOSU career.

Rest assured! The wobbling is normal—and may even help you learn something about your body. As you wobble, try to notice what is going on in your body. Where are the adjustments taking place: in your feet, your knees, your hips? Are there any patterns, such as placing more weight on one foot or the other, or a tendency to move toward one side of the dome? If you notice a pattern, is there something you can do to offset it? In other words, is there something you can consciously do to help your body learn how to balance better? What about your head and eyes? Try to avoid looking down. Looking straight ahead helps your eyes and your body stabilize.

Whether you notice a pattern or not, the more you practice, the less you'll wobble because the nervous system gets better at making the appropriate neuromuscular adjustments. With time, you'll become stronger and more secure and you'll be able to stand and move on the BOSU with greater confidence and stability.

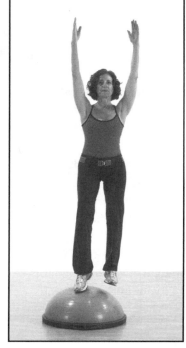

the core of the matter

These days it seems that everybody is talking about core strength and stability. Many people think that the core is synonymous with the abs. Not so! The abs are only a part of the core. The full core extends from the upper torso and neck to the knees, and serves as a link between the upper and lower body.

According to the Mayo Clinic website, there are as many as 29 core muscles within the trunk and pelvis. In practice, most trainers and sports practitioners focus on a subsection of this group of muscles and include the following as part of the core:

- the deeper abdominals (transversus abdominis, internal and external obliques) and pelvic floor
- gluteals and hamstrings
- back muscles (multifidus muscles, quadratus lumborum, serratus anterior, latissimus dorsi, erector spinae)

Stuart McGill, Ph.D., a leading Canadian expert on lower back problems, concurs. He suggests that many trunk muscles, abdominals, and back muscles contribute to stabilization. Sometimes we put too much emphasis on one muscle, thinking it's more important than others. McGill believes that many muscles work together to build a strong back and strengthen the core.

When we work out on the BOSU, we train two types of muscles: mobilizers and stabilizers. Mobilizers are usually larger, more superficial muscles. They're designed for short, powerful movements. Our gluteals ("glutes") are a good example. Stabilizers, also known as core muscles, pro-

vide support during movement and are typically deeper and smaller. Examples include the deep abdominal muscles as well as the small muscles around the shoulder blades, which help position the arm correctly in the socket. Because the BOSU requires a lot of balance, we're particularly interested in our core muscles.

Abdominal muscles

There are four abdominal muscles ("abs"): transversus abdominis, the internal and external obliques, and the rectus abdominis.

The transversus abdominis is the deepest and one of the

most important muscles of the core. As the name implies, it goes around the body; its fibers run horizontally around the waist. Together with the multifidus muscles, it helps to stabilize the lower spine by narrowing the abdominal wall when it's contracted.

The internal and external obliques play a significant role in stabilizing the hips and rib cage and connecting the upper and lower body. They're also responsible for side-bending and twisting the spine.

The rectus abdominis is the most superficial of the abs. It runs up from the pubic bone to the sternum and helps us bend forward.

Pelvic floor muscles

Also known as Kegel muscles, the pelvic floor is another important core muscle for both men and women. Running from front to back at the base of the pelvis, it looks and acts like a sling, holding our lower inner organs. The pelvic floor muscles connect through the nervous system to the deep abdominals.

Finding the pelvic floor muscles can be elusive. Some people find it helpful to imagine they have a very full bladder and are trying to stop the flow of urine as they search for a bathroom. The idea is to feel the pelvic floor

muscles gently squeeze together as the bottom of the pelvis draws up.

By tightening, or pulling up on, the pelvic floor you also connect to your deeper abdominals and indirectly to some of the core muscles in your back, helping you to stabilize and stay connected.

Deep back muscles

The deep back muscles consist primarily of the erector spinae, multifidus muscles, and the quadratus lumborum (QL). The latter two are key back stabilizers.

The multifidus muscles are some of the deepest back extensors. They consist of small bundles that pass from one vertebra to another and have been shown to activate the deep abdominal muscles. Together they help stabilize the spine.

The quadratus lumborum runs vertically and connects the lower back with the ribs and pelvis. It therefore plays a role in connecting and stabilizing the upper and lower body as we move. This muscle also helps us bend to the side.

Back and buttock muscles

Our trapezius, or "trap" muscles, start at the neck and extend to the middle of our back on both sides. We use

them primarily to move our shoulders. The latissimus dorsi ("lats") are large, broad muscles that extend from our lower and mid-back on each side, wrap around our torso, and insert on our upper arms. These muscles play a role in stabilizing our shoulders and in some arm movements.

Taken together, our gluteals ("glutes") help us move but also stabilize the pelvis when we walk or move our legs. There are three glute muscles: gluteus maximus, the biggest "prime mover" in the body; gluteus medius, a smaller but very significant stabilizing muscle; and the gluteus minimus. The gluteus maximus is one of the strongest muscles in the body. It's a major hip extensor and also helps to rotate the leg outward. While smaller, the gluteus medius plays a big role in supporting the hips when we stand and move and is often associated with postural problems. The gluteus minimus helps with bending, lifting, and rotating the femur in the hip socket.

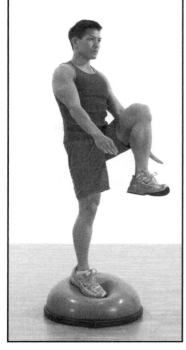

it's all about U

To help people visualize the muscles in the core, some fitness industry specialists talk about the serape effect (referring to the Mexican shawl), which consists of the rhomboids, serratus anterior, and external and internal obliques. The idea is that these muscles work together as connectors and stabilizers.

The serape effect also explains the cross-connection between opposite sides of the body and how, for example, focusing on the connection between our shoulder and opposite hip or knee helps us balance when we lift one leg or step or lunge forward onto the BOSU on one foot.

Pilates practitioners have similar ways of characterizing the core muscles. Some talk about using the powerhouse (the area between the bottom rib and the pelvis, the lower back and the buttocks). Joseph Pilates himself referred to this area as a "girdle of strength" and believed that initiating

movement from the core helped one move safely and efficiently. Others use the image of a corset (the band of muscles encircling the torso and extending from the lower rib cage to just below the buttocks).

Carolyn Richardson and her associates, Australian authorities on spinal stabilization, describe the core muscles as a three-dimensional cylinder (from the pelvic floor on the bottom to the diaphragm on top and from the transversus abdominis in front and on the sides, to the multifidus muscles in the back). When contracted, these muscles transform the abdomen and

spine into a rigid cylinder.

Another analogy focuses on the "U," an imaginary smile from hip to hip, formed in the abdomen by engaging the Kegel or pelvic floor muscles along with the transversus and obliques. Using this approach, practitioners pull up their pelvic floor and draw in the low belly between the pubic bone and navel (sometimes cued as pulling up one's zipper muscles). The goal is to feel the pelvic floor muscles gently squeeze together as the bottom of the pelvis draws up, which helps lift the internal organs and engage the transversus. At the same time, drawing the rib

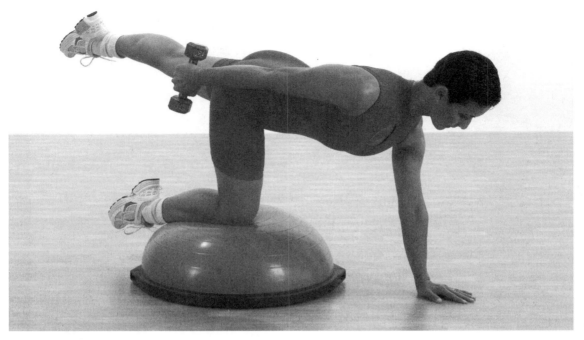

cage toward the hip (think of the dimples in the smile) activates the internal obliques that stabilize the hips.

These approaches have one thing in common. They all focus on finding and strengthening the muscles that protect and brace the spine, torso, and pelvis so that we have a solid base from which to move with strength and ease. The main message is that core strength and stability are the keys to successful movement. Getting there is what's important. The cue or image used to get there is secondary.

Brace yourself

When we talk about the core muscles contracting and stabi- lizing the spine, it almost sounds like they turn on by themselves. However, their performance is not entirely automatic—at least not initially. Like any muscle or group of muscles, the core muscles must be trained.

Ultimately, the goal is to have our core muscles respond without consciously calling them to action. But at first, and for some time, we must actively recruit these muscles to stabilize our spines and help us move safely and effectively.

In other words, we have to learn to "brace ourselves" or engage our core muscles before we do certain moves. Stuart McGill describes bracing as "stiffening the abdominal wall." In a February 2007 *New York Times* article, he empha- sized that "it's not sucking in and it's not pushing your belly out." Instead, he advises, "Pretend you are going to get whacked in the belly." While this bracing action is not iden- tical to the methods described above, the same muscles are involved and the outcome is similar—moving from a place of strength and stability.

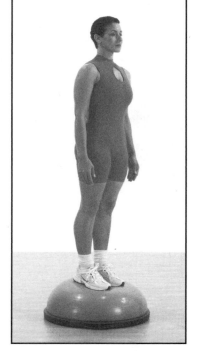

starting in neutral

Successful movement depends on good alignment, and the foundation of good alignment is a neutral spine. A neutral spine is one where the natural spinal curves are present. When viewed from the side, a neutral spine typically has four curves:

- a slight inward curve at the neck (called the cervical spine)
- an outward curve at the top of the ribs (called the thoracic spine)
- a more pronounced inward curve at the small of the back (called the lumbar spine)
- a small outward curve at the base of the spine

These curves are desirable because they protect and minimize the amount of stress on the spine and surrounding tissue by absorbing shock when we move. Put another way, "Neutral alignment allows the joints and muscles to perform at their best with the least risk of injury" (*Elphinston and Pook, p. 16*).

Finding neutral

To find your body's "neutral" position, stand with a slight bend in your knees and hips. With your hip bones pointing forward like the headlights of a car, slowly tilt your pelvis forward so your lower back rounds into a slight tuck. Then tilt your pelvis backward so your lower back is in a slight arch. The point between the tuck and the arch is your body's neutral position.

You can also find neutral by lying down on your back with your knees bent and feet flat on the floor. There should be two places where your spine does not touch the floor: under your neck and under your lower back. At this point, your spine is in a neutral position.

Is that all there is?

Finding your neutral spine is not the end of the story. Even with all the curves intact, your spine doesn't just sit there by itself. The long, superficial muscles of the trunk, together with the smaller, deeper muscles in the abdomen and back that act to support and stabilize the individual bones of the spine, hold the spine in place.

Many people liken the spine to a multisegmented flagpole, with the large, superficial back muscles acting like the guy wires that balance the flagpole and the smaller, deeper muscles acting like the

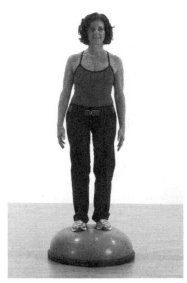

Neutral spine

links that keep each segment of the pole together and erect. In body terms, the larger, superficial muscles are involved with large, dynamic movements, such as arching or bending the trunk; the smaller, deeper abdominal and back muscles help stabilize the spine and keep the body upright. If the deep muscles are weak or don't work effectively, the back may become unstable and other muscles may be called on to fill in or compensate.

The point is that correct alignment—not only in the spine but in the whole body—makes the right muscles available and provides the opportunity for them to work properly. Moreover, finding a neutral spine is only part of the whole alignment story. Think of a plumb line moving from the very top of your head through your body to your feet. Your collar bones are wide, your shoulders and chest are open, your arms hang naturally and comfortably by your sides. Your spine is in neutral. Your feet are hip-width apart (right under your hip bones), your feet are parallel. You are at rest, standing up. There is no stress on any part of your body.

This is what optimal body alignment is all about. The goal is to maintain this stress-free state when you exercise. This doesn't mean you won't be engaging muscles and working your body. But you'll be doing so without additional stress caused by incorrect positioning or overusing the wrong muscles.

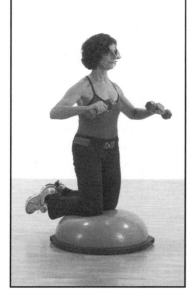

practicing safe BOSU

One of the neat things about the BOSU is that it's very easy to mount and dismount. So if you lose your balance at any point, simply step off and start over when you're ready. As with any piece of exercise equipment, however, it pays to be careful. The following tips will help make your BOSU experience safer and more rewarding.

Inflate your BOSU correctly. Follow the instructions that came with your dome.

Place your BOSU on a level surface like a wood floor or carpet. Consider using a mat for exercises where knees or other bony parts touch the floor. A mat also keeps the BOSU from slipping. Be sure you have plenty of space around you.

Wear shoes when you work out on the BOSU. Shoes protect your feet and add support, particularly when you step onto and off of the dome. A good athletic shoe like a cross-trainer is recommended. Do not wear street shoes as they may transfer grit to the surface of the dome and possibly damage it.

Note: Some people prefer to work with bare feet for moves that don't require stepping onto and off of the dome. Working barefoot can be both challenging and strengthening, particularly for your ankles and arches. However, you should never work in stocking feet because you could slip and hurt yourself.

Use a towel to wipe your dome dry as needed to keep from slipping and falling.

Keep a set of hand weights nearby. While all exercises can be done without weights, adding resistance not only strengthens targeted muscles, it also challenges your balance and core stability.

Use props. If you feel unstable at any time, use a body bar, broomstick, or the wall for additional support.

Work at your own pace and level. Know your limits and keep the workout safe. Remember that you can step off the dome any time you feel unstable or unsafe and get back on when you regain your balance.

Aim for 2–3 workouts per week of at least 20–30 minutes each.

DON'T HOLD YOUR BREATH!

Breathing. It comes naturally, right? Yes, at least to some extent. But it can be so much more!

It may surprise you to learn that many people hold their breath, or breathe shallowly at best, especially when they exercise. Often we are so preoccupied that we forget all about breathing!

Without breath, our muscles and organs would starve. Literally! Breathing pumps oxygen—and all kinds of nutrients and energy—throughout our bodies. The deeper we breathe, the more we nourish our insides.

The moral of the story? Work your breath just like you work your body. Inhale deeply through the nose to prepare for each exercise, and exhale deeply through your mouth on the exertion. Aside from ridding your body of unwanted waste, exhaling—especially exhaling audibly and with some force through your mouth—helps engage the core, and the abs in particular.

People often feel self-conscious making noise as they breathe. Instead, think about the benefits of connecting your breath to your work. Breathe with intention. It focuses your effort both physically and mentally.

Breathe life into your BOSU workouts! And enjoy all the benefits that they bring.

can use the flat side for push-ups, bridge exercises, and other moves.

- Never exercise on a full stomach.
- Read all the exercise instructions thoroughly before you begin and pay attention to any tips and modifications.

Other safety tips

- Check with your health practitioner or doctor before you start to make sure the exercises are suitable for you. If in doubt about individual exercises, avoid them until you get professional advice.
- Standing on the platform side of the BOSU is not recommended. However, you

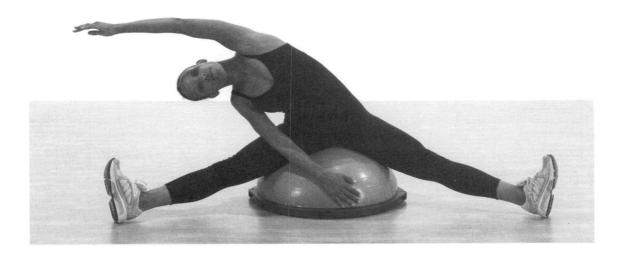

part 2:
BOSU
basics

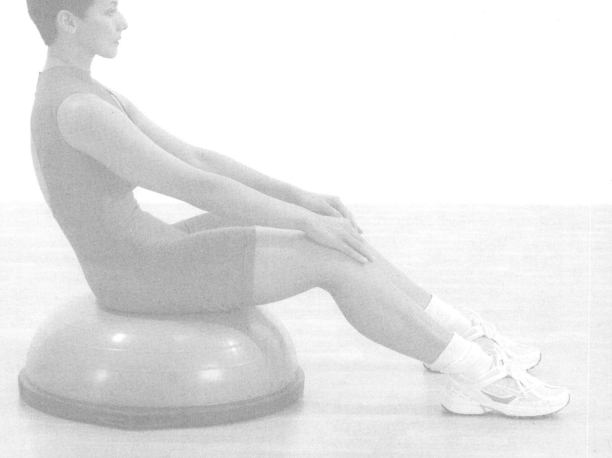

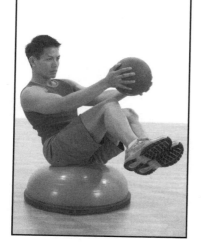

getting started

To set out on our BOSU journey, we start with some simpler moves, including standing and balancing on the dome. The exercises are aimed at those who have never worked on a BOSU before, but they're also a great warm-up and reminder for experienced enthusiasts. This section of the book contains basic repertoire that forms a foundation for the selections that appear later.

One of the first challenges on the BOSU has to do with foot placement. We're used to standing on a flat surface. Thus, when we first step onto the BOSU, our feet tend to conform to the rounded shape of the dome, which means our feet are not level. If our feet aren't level, our muscles aren't aligned properly. That makes it harder to balance. And without balance, it's difficult to stand or move from a stable base.

For this reason, working out on the BOSU is all about teaching—or reminding—our bodies about balance and sta-bility on the unstable surface of the dome. Throughout the exercises, therefore, we strive for level feet, good alignment, and correct placement so we are in the best position (liter-ally) to develop and train our muscles.

With this in mind, and before we proceed, here are some general guidelines for working out on the BOSU:

- Place your feet about hip-width apart on either side of the bull's eye.
- Bend your knees slightly and make sure your toes point forward.

- Stand with a neutral spine and look straight ahead (looking down can throw you off balance). Imagine a plumb line descending from the top of your head and ending between your feet.
- Make sure your shoulders are relaxed (not up at your ears!) and that your head is in line with your spine.
- Keep your hips facing forward and your knees in line with your toes.
- Press firmly on the insides of your feet

to engage your adductors (or inner thighs).

- Engage your core muscles. They stabilize your spine, pelvis, and shoulders and keep your upper and lower body connected.
- Breathe! Exhale audibly through your mouth to help you connect to your core, especially your abs. Above all, don't hold your breath!

The rest of Part 2 introduces several basic exercises in a variety of positions, many of which reappear as part of later selections. If you're new to the BOSU, you may want to take your time and get comfortable with the moves in this section before you proceed.

Note: You will notice that several of the exercises start by telling you to stand a "comfortable" distance behind or beside the BOSU. Because body proportions differ, there is no fixed starting position. For example, if you have long legs, you will stand further back than someone with shorter legs. You may, therefore, have to experiment to find your best starting position.

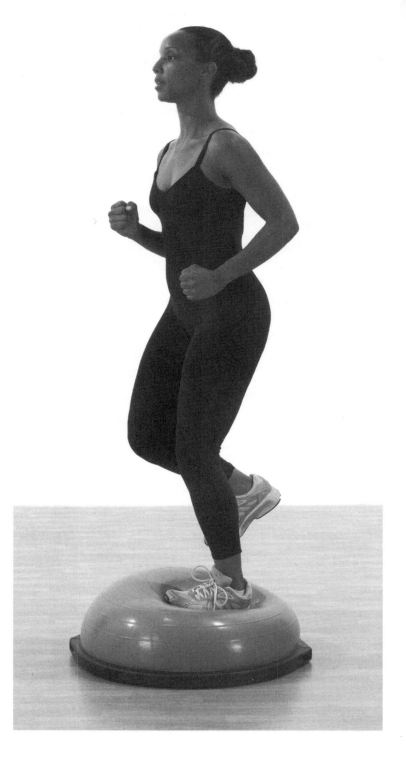

moving on and off the dome

The exercises in this section will help you become accustomed to moving between the floor and the dome. They involve transferring your weight and adjusting to the differences between the stability of the floor and the instability of the BOSU.

Helpful hints
- Make sure your ankles don't roll in or out.
- Keep your knees over your toes.
- Relax your shoulders and reach tall through the crown of your head.

- Look straight ahead (looking down can throw you off balance).

stepping up and down

STARTING POSITION: Stand a comfortable distance behind the dome with your feet about hip-width apart. Rest your hands by your sides.

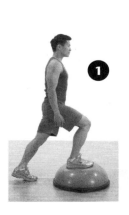
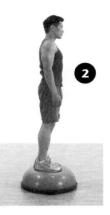
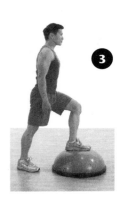

starting position

1 Slowly step onto the dome with your right foot, aiming just to the right of the bull's eye.

2 Slowly step onto the dome with your left foot so that your feet end up on either side of the bull's eye.

3 Dismount by stepping back off the dome with your right foot, followed by your left foot.

Repeat 4–5 times, then start over on the other side.

TIPS
- Keep your shoulders and hips facing forward.
- Step firmly onto the top of the dome.
- Aim to land on either side of the bull's eye.

STARTING POSITION: Stand a comfortable distance behind the dome. Raise your arms in front of you.

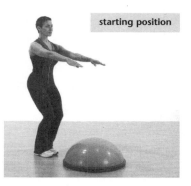

starting position

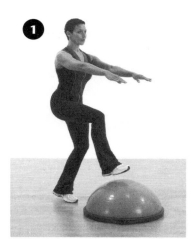

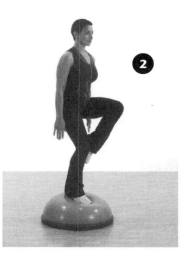

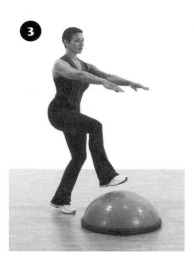

1 Step onto the dome with your right foot, aiming for the bull's eye.

2 Lean slightly forward. At the same time, bend your left leg and lift your knee toward your body.

3 Dismount by stepping back to the floor behind the dome with your left foot, followed by your right foot.

Start over on the other side. Then alternate from side to side.

Repeat 4–5 times.

TIPS

• Plant your foot firmly on the dome. Aim for the bull's eye each time.

building balance and stability

When you first stand on the dome, your body may wobble as it adjusts to the unstable surface of the dome. With practice, your brain and body learn how to adapt to the new surface.

When you stand on the dome, remember to keep your pelvis and spine in "neutral"— their safest and most natural position. Also remember to engage your core. These muscles help you stay connected and erect.

Helpful hints
- Engage your abs to connect to your core and create a strong center.
- Look straight ahead and keep your neck long. The position of your head affects your balance.

standing on the dome

STARTING POSITION: Stand a comfortable distance behind the dome. Rest your hands by your sides.

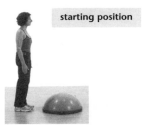
starting position

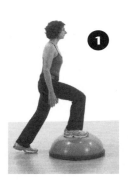
1

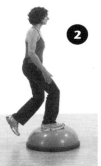
2

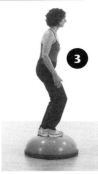
3

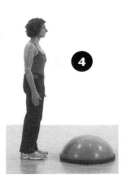
4

1 Slowly step onto the dome with your right foot.

2 Slowly step onto the dome with your left foot.

3 Stand with your knees slightly bent and your spine in a neutral position. Hold for 5 counts.

4 Step back to your starting position.

TIPS
- Keep your knees over your toes.
- Avoid tucking your pelvis. Let your tailbone be heavy.
- Make sure your feet are level.

CHALLENGE
Stand on the dome with your eyes closed. It's much harder this way because there are no visual cues for the brain to use.

STARTING POSITION: Stand on the dome with your knees bent and your feet level and about hip-width apart. Hold your arms out to the sides in a T.

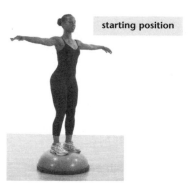

starting position

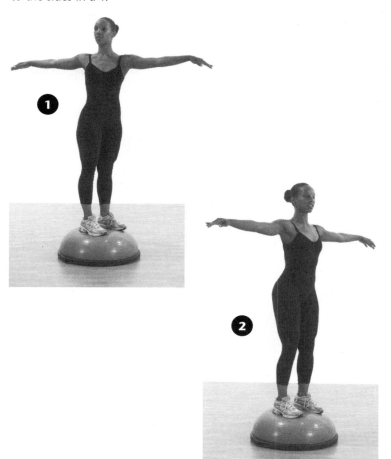

1

2

1 Keeping your hips square and facing forward, lift out of your hips and twist from your waist to the right.

2 Twist back to center.

Repeat 4–5 times, then start over on the other side.

SUPER CHALLENGE

Hold a weighted ball in front of your torso as you twist. Keep your wrists strong and aligned with your forearms.

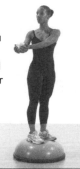

TIPS

• Relax your shoulders and keep your head in line with your spine.

kneeling on the dome

Kneeling on the dome can be tricky because your vertical center of gravity changes. This means that your brain has to adjust to a new pattern of weight distribution. You may be surprised at how quickly you can adapt!

Caution: Avoid all kneeling exercises if you have knee issues.

kneeling tall

STARTING POSITION: Kneel on the dome with one knee on each side of the bull's eye. Rest your toes on the floor behind you. Hold your arms out to the sides in a T.

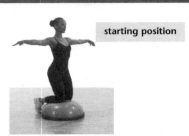

starting position

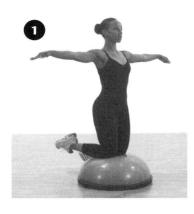

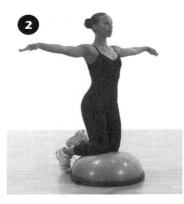

1 Engage your core and lift the toes of one foot off the floor. Hold for 5 counts and release.

2 Lift the toes of the other foot off the floor. Hold for 5 counts and release.

3 Staying centered over your knees with even weight on both knees, lift the toes of both feet off the floor. Hold for 5 counts and release.

Repeat 4–5 times.

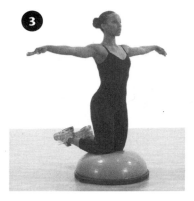

TIPS

- Reach the crown of your head toward the ceiling throughout the exercise.
- Engage your lower abs and inner thighs to stay connected and tall.

kneeling

kneeling on all fours

STARTING POSITION: Kneel on all fours with your knees about hip-width apart on the dome. Place your hands on the floor in front of the dome.

starting position

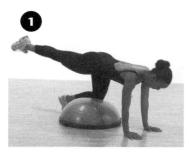

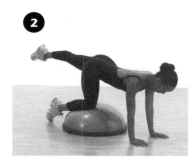

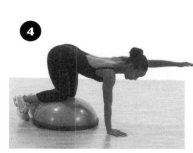

1 Engage your core and slowly lift and extend your right leg behind you to hip height. Then lower it back down.

2 Stay connected and slowly lift and extend your left leg behind you to hip height. Then lower it back down.

3 Focus on your lower abs and slowly lift and extend your right arm in front of you to shoulder height. Then lower it back down.

4 Stay connected and slowly lift and extend your left arm in front of you to shoulder height. Then lower it back down.

Repeat 4–5 times.

TIPS

- Press firmly from the heels of your hands to avoid sinking between your shoulder blades.
- Make sure your knees and hips are level and face forward.
- Keep your neck long and your head in line with your spine.

CHALLENGE

Extend your opposite leg and arm at the same time.

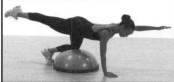

working the abs, hamstrings, and glutes

Without the support of the core, we have trouble with more challenging moves.

The exercises in this section focus on your abs, hamstrings, and glutes. They help you

build your core and form a strong foundation for later exercises.

pelvic tilt

Caution: If you have a sensitive lower back, keep the tilting movements small. Avoid over-arching or over-flattening your back.

STARTING POSITION: Sit on the dome with your hips on the bull's eye. Place your feet hip-width apart and flat on the floor and your hands on your knees.

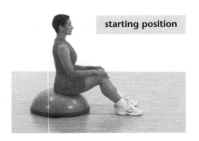

starting position

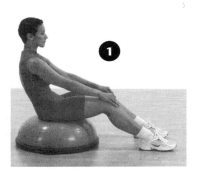

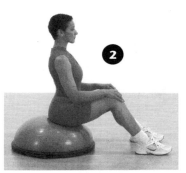

1 Contract your lower abs to curl your pelvis forward, flattening your lower back. Hold for 2 counts and release.

2 Slowly tilt your pelvis backward so your lower back is arched. Hold for 2 counts and release.

Repeat 4–5 times, building some speed as you go.

TIPS
- Keep your upper body still as you move your pelvis.
- Use your lower abs, not your glutes, to move your pelvis back and forth.

hip roll in bridge

STARTING POSITION: Sit on the floor with your back facing the dome and your lower back resting gently against the front edge of the BOSU. Bend your knees and place your feet flat on the floor. Rest your hands on the floor next to your hips.

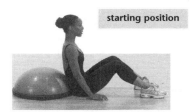

starting position

1

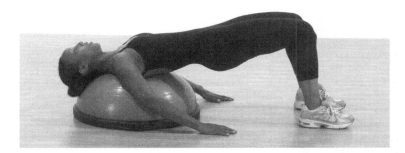

1 Press into your feet and slowly lift your hips off the floor, one vertebra at a time, until your upper back, shoulders, and head rest on the dome.

2 Slowly roll back down one vertebra at a time to your starting position.

Repeat 4–5 times.

2

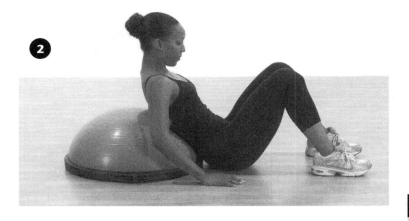

TIPS

- Make sure you're centered on the dome.
- Press into your feet throughout the exercise to keep your hips lifted and stay connected to your core.

working the back and legs

In this section, you'll be working face-down on the dome and be asked to extend either your spine or a limb. Moving a part of your body away from its center will place a signifi-cant demand on your core. To protect your back, be sure to engage your lower belly.

Because we all have different body proportions, you may have to adjust your position on the dome to find your center of gravity. For more information, see page 25.

single-leg extension

STARTING POSITION: Lie face-down with your torso on top of the dome. Extend your legs straight out behind you. Rest your hands on the floor in front of the dome. *Note:* Adjust your position to find your center of gravity.

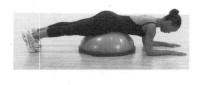

starting position

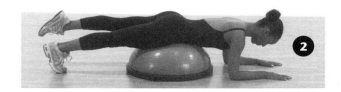

1 Lifting from your glutes, not your back, extend and lift your right leg no higher than hip height. Hold for 2 counts, then lower your leg back down.

2 Extend and lift your left leg no higher than hip height. Hold for 2 counts, then lower it back down.

Repeat 4–5 times.

CHALLENGE
Lift the opposite arm and leg at the same time. Hold for 5 counts.

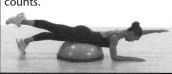

TIPS
• Keep your head in line with your spine throughout the exercise.

STARTING POSITION: Lie face-down with your torso on top of the dome, keeping your legs bent or straight. Extend your arms back toward your hips and rest your palms on top of the dome. Keep your head relaxed. *Note:* Adjust your position to find your center of gravity.

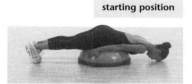

starting position

1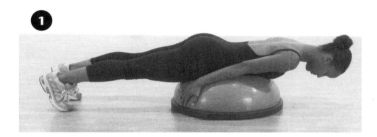

1 Engage your lower abs and, keeping your neck long, hover your head just above the floor.

2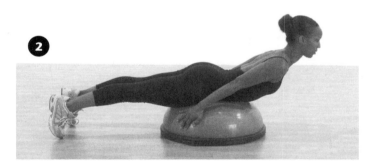

2 Leading with the crown of your head, slowly peel your upper body off the dome as far as you can without arching your lower back. Avoid crunching your upper back and neck. Hold for 2 counts.

3 Slowly release back to your starting position.

Repeat 4–5 times.

3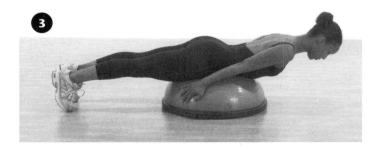

TIPS

- Keep your head in line with your spine throughout the exercise.
- Extend out of your hips to lengthen your back.

working with squats and lunges

Squats and lunges work the hamstrings, glutes, and quads, but can't be done without help from the abs and other core muscles. The BOSU forces you to work in an integrated and functional way. The stronger your core, the better you will perform—on and off the BOSU.

squatting on the dome

STARTING POSITION: Stand on the dome with your knees bent and your feet level and about hip-width apart. Rest your hands by your sides.

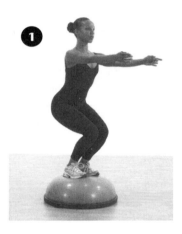

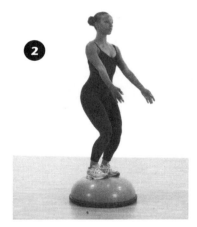

starting position

1 Slowly bend your knees into a squat, keeping your back flat and your knees over your toes. At the same time, arc your arms straight out in front of you. Hold for 2 counts.

2 Slowly straighten up to your starting position, lowering your arms back down by your sides.

Repeat 4–5 times.

TIPS

• Make sure your head is in line with your spine throughout the exercise.
• Engage your lower abs and inner thighs for stability.
• Avoid arching or tucking your pelvis.

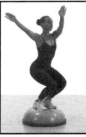

CHALLENGE

Circle your arms in front of you as you squat. Start at the top and circle toward the right. For even more challenge, follow your arms with your eyes. Looking overhead is especially tricky!

STARTING POSITION: Stand on the dome with your knees bent and your feet level and about hip-width apart. Hold your hands in front of your torso and bend your elbows.

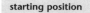
starting position

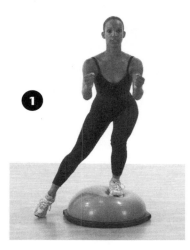

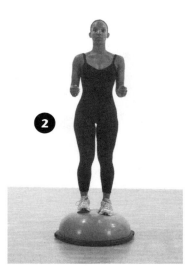

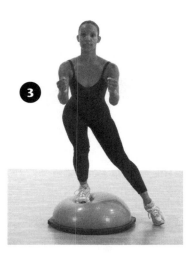

1 Lean forward slightly from your hips (as if you were in a slight squat) and tap your right toes on the floor to the right of the dome.

2 Step back onto the dome with your right foot.

3 Repeat steps 1–2 to the left.

Repeat several times.

TIPS

• Stay centered and low over the dome. The more compact you are, the easier it is to move.
• Engage your inner thighs and lower abs for stability.

CHALLENGE

Gradually add speed and, as you lunge, move your arms in opposition to your body to off-set the weight shift.

leaving the surface of the dome

Jumps are especially challenging on the dome, but they're fun and also good for you because they build bone mass.

Fortunately, the surface of the BOSU has some "give" and softens the shock of a jump. At the same time, the instability of the surface can throw you off and forces the body to adjust.

stepping on top of the dome

STARTING POSITION: Stand on the dome with your knees bent and your feet level and about hip-width apart. Rest your hands by your sides.

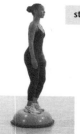
starting position

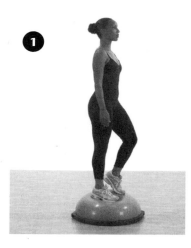
1

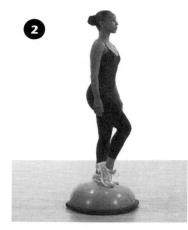
2

1 Transfer your weight to your right foot and slowly step onto your right foot. Hold for 2 counts.

2 Transfer your weight to your left foot and slowly step onto your left foot. Hold for 2 counts.

Repeat several times.

CHALLENGE
Change to a more deliberate march. Then try raising your knees high as you march.

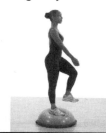

SUPER CHALLENGE
Speed up to a jog.

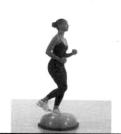

TIPS
- Place your feet on either side of the bull's eye as you transfer your weight from side to side.
- Face forward and focus on a point in front of you.
- Engage your core to stay connected from head to toe.

STARTING POSITION: Stand a comfortable distance behind the dome. Rest your hands by your sides.

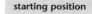
starting position

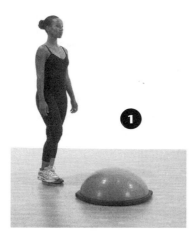

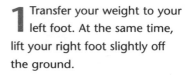

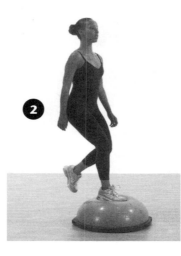

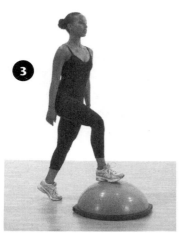

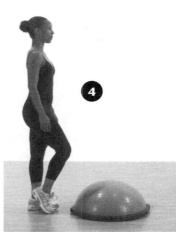

1 Transfer your weight to your left foot. At the same time, lift your right foot slightly off the ground.

2 Jump onto the dome with your right foot, aiming for the bull's eye. Land firmly on a bent knee.

3 Step back off the dome with your left foot.

4 Tap your right foot lightly beside your left foot.

Repeat 4–5 times, then start over on the other side.

TIPS

- Plant your foot firmly on the dome to "stick" your landing.
- Engage your abs and brace your shoulders to stay connected.

single-foot sideways jump

STARTING POSITION: Stand a comfortable distance to the left of the dome. Rest your hands by your sides.

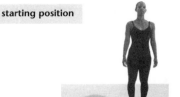

starting position

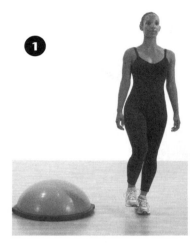

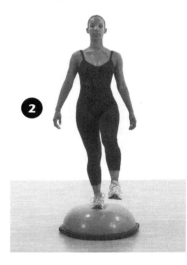

1 Transfer your weight to your left foot. At the same time, lift your right foot slightly off the ground.

2 Jump onto the dome with your right foot, aiming for the bull's eye. Land firmly on a bent knee.

3 Step back off the dome with your left foot.

4 Tap your right foot lightly on the floor beside your left foot.

Repeat 4–5 times, then start over on the other side.

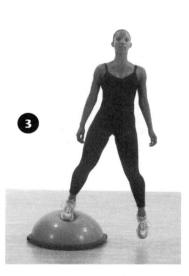

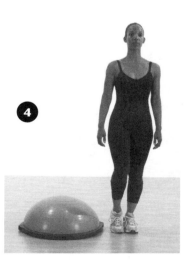

TIPS

- Plant your foot firmly on the dome to "stick" your landing.
- Engage your abs and brace your shoulders to stay connected.

part 3:
the
exercises

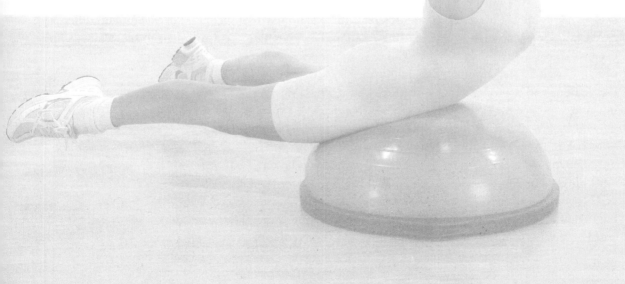

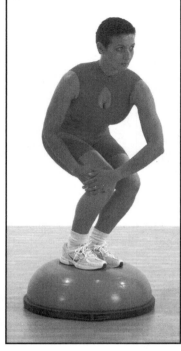

about the exercises

Part 3 contains several exercises grouped by exercise type: squats, lunges, back exercises, and so on. Because most BOSU exercises work more than one muscle group at a time, the exercises are loosely grouped—more for organizational purposes than anything else.

Each exercise category starts with a brief introduction and a list of *Helpful hints*. Please read these closely and follow them for your own safety and enjoyment. If you've had an injury, consult your medical practitioner to make sure the exercises are suitable for you.

Within a category, each exercise shows a starting position, followed by step-by-step instructions and plenty of illustrative photos for each move. Please read the instructions before you start.

Following most exercises is a list of relevant *Tips*—ideas to keep in mind or cues to improve the execution. There are also variations of the main

exercise—*Basic*, *Challenge*, and *Super Challenge*—to accommodate different fitness levels.

Note: Several exercises start by telling you to stand a "comfortable" distance behind or beside the BOSU. Because everyone's body proportions are different, there is no fixed starting position. For example, if your legs are longer, you'll stand further back than someone with shorter legs. You may, therefore, have to experiment to find your best starting position.

Similarly when you lie on the dome, whether it's face-down, face-up, or sideways, you may have to adjust your position to find your center of

gravity. If your legs are relatively longer than the rest of your body, you'll probably feel more balanced if the bull's eye is closer to your head. If your torso is relatively longer than the rest of your body, the reverse will probably suit you better. Experiment with different positions to see what works best.

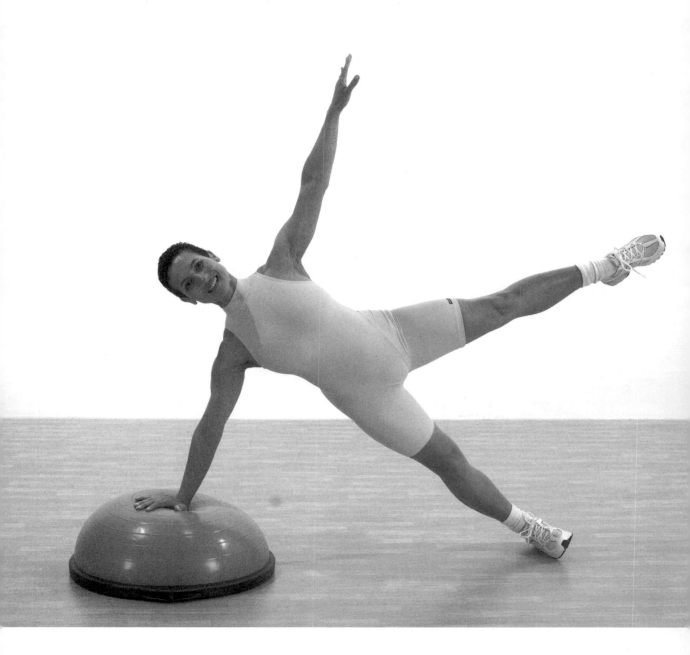

cardio and jumps

Cardio is short for cardiovascular. Cardio exercises pump up the heart rate, expand lung capacity, and improve circulation. Other benefits include weight loss, increased bone density, improved health, more energy, and sounder sleep.

Using the BOSU for cardio is a lot like using an aerobics step. You can use similar patterns and combinations as well as music to energize and enhance your workouts.

This section introduces some of these moves and also includes a series of jumps. It takes a lot of balance, control, and stability to land jumps on a level surface. Landing on the rounded dome of a BOSU makes the task even more daunting, but it can also be a lot of fun.

The surface of the BOSU cushions your body as you jump on it, but it can also throw you off balance. Many people make the mistake of trying to jump too high. Take your time and start small so that your body can adjust to the surface and you can gain more control.

Helpful hints

- Practice on the floor first to get used to the pattern.
- Connect to your core and brace yourself from head to toe.
- Keep your knees bent and inner thighs strong.
- Land firmly on top of the dome with both feet flat and level.
- Spread the weight through your whole foot to help you balance. Avoid rolling in or out.
- Face forward, make sure your hips and shoulders are square, and look straight ahead.
- Exhale audibly through your mouth, especially on exertion, to connect to your core and help you through those extra-challenging moments.

STARTING POSITION: Stand a comfortable distance behind the dome with your knees slightly bent. Extend your arms in front of you at shoulder height.

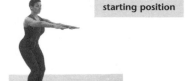

starting position

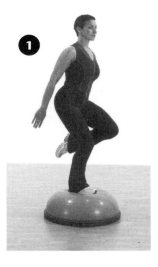

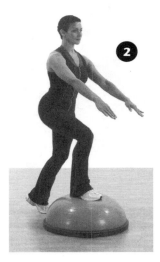

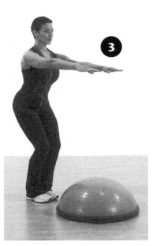

1 Leap firmly onto the dome with your right foot, aiming for the bull's eye. As you land, exhale to connect to your core and make sure your supporting knee is bent; swing your arms backward. Hold for 2 counts.

2 Dismount by stepping back off the dome with your left foot. At the same time swing your arms forward.

3 Step your right foot back to join your left, keeping your arms forward.

Start over on the other side after your right foot touches back. Then alternate from side to side.

Repeat 4–5 times.

Count	1	2	3	4
Cue	Leap	Hold	Back	Step

STARTING POSITION: Stand a comfortable distance behind the dome with your hips, knees, and toes facing forward. Rest your hands by your sides.

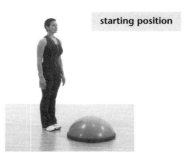

starting position

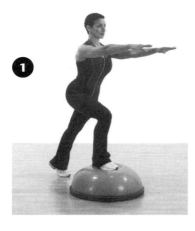

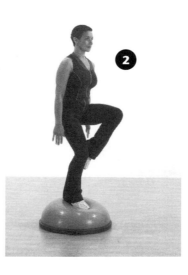

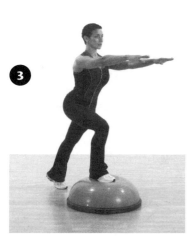

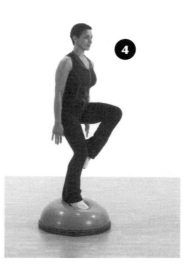

1 Step firmly onto the bull's eye with your right foot, leaning slightly forward as you plant your foot. At the same time, swing your arms forward to shoulder height.

2 Bend your left knee in toward your body. At the same time, swing your arms backward.

3 Straighten your left leg behind you and tap your toe on the floor. At the same time, swing your arms forward.

4 Repeat steps 2 and 3 again. Then bend your left knee in toward your chest one more time, swinging your arms backward.

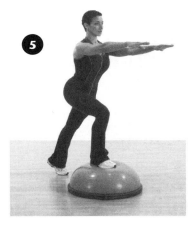

TIPS

- Stay low as you move.
- Contract your abs, especially your low belly, to help you stabilize.

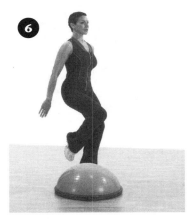

5 Dismount by stepping back off the dome with your left foot. At the same time, swing your arms forward.

6 Step your right foot back to join your left and swing your arms backward.

Start over on the other side after your right foot touches back. Then alternate from side to side.

Repeat 4–5 times.

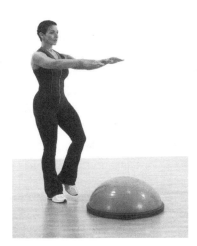

Count	1	2	3	4	5	6	7	8
Cue	Step	Knee	Straighten	Knee	Straighten	Knee	Back	Step

STARTING POSITION: Stand a comfortable distance behind the dome with your hips, knees, and toes facing forward. Rest your hands by your sides.

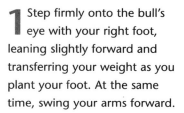

starting position

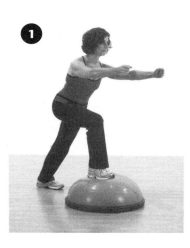

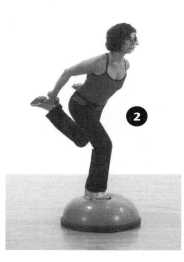

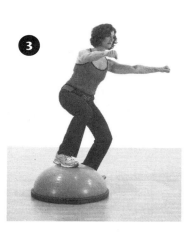

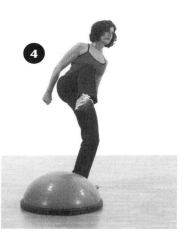

1 Step firmly onto the bull's eye with your right foot, leaning slightly forward and transferring your weight as you plant your foot. At the same time, swing your arms forward.

2 Bend your left knee and lift your leg behind you in a leg curl. At the same time, swing your arms backward.

3 Step your left foot down onto the floor to the left of the dome. At the same time, swing your arms forward.

4 Leaning slightly to the left, lift your right leg and bend your right knee in toward your chest. At the same time, swing your arms backward.

5 Step back onto the dome with your right foot. At the same time, swing your arms forward.

6 Lift your left leg behind you in a leg curl again. At the same time, swing your arms backward.

7 Dismount by stepping back off the dome with your left foot. At the same time, swing your arms forward.

8 Step your right foot back to join your left and swing your arms backward.

Start over on the other side after your right foot touches back. Then alternate from side to side.

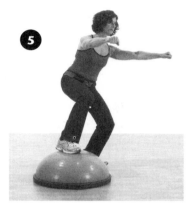

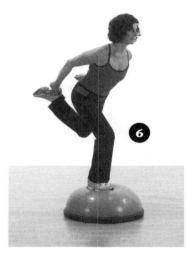

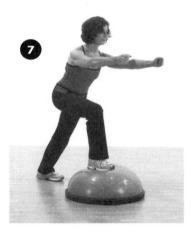

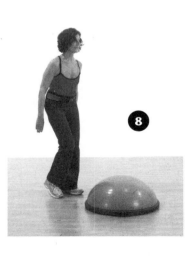

TIPS

- Stay centered over your hips as you move.
- Keep your shoulders and hips facing forward.
- Contract your abs, especially your low belly, to help you stabilize.

Count	1	2	3	4	5	6	7	8
Cue	Step	Curl	Step	Lift	Step	Curl	Back	Step

STARTING POSITION: Stand a comfortable distance behind the dome with your hips, knees, and toes facing forward. Rest your hands by your sides.

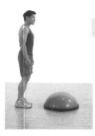

starting position

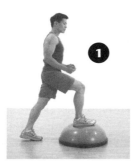

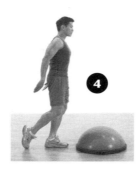

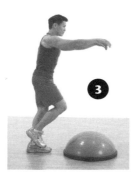

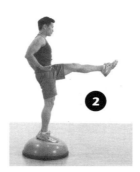

1 Step firmly onto the bull's eye with your right foot. At the same time, swing your arms forward.

2 Bend your left knee and kick your foot out in front of you. At the same time, draw your elbows in to your waist and make fists with your hands.

3 Dismount by stepping back off the dome with your left foot while reaching your arms straight out in front of you.

4 Tap back with your right foot and swing your arms backward.

Repeat 4–5 times, then start over on the other side.

SUPER CHALLENGE

Alternate between kicking the left foot forward and reaching it back as you lunge, keeping the back leg straight.

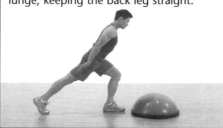

Count	1	2	3	4
Cue	Step	Kick	Back	Step

TIPS

- Keep your shoulders and hips facing forward.
- Avoid leaning forward or backward as you kick.

STARTING POSITION: Stand a comfortable distance to the left of the dome with your feet about hip-width apart and your hips, knees, and toes facing forward. Rest your hands by your sides.

starting position

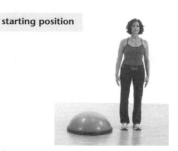

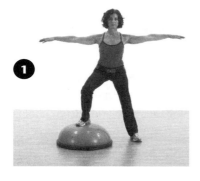

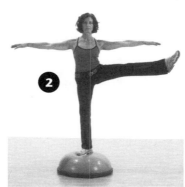

1 Step firmly onto the dome with your right foot and lift your arms to a T.

2 Keeping both legs straight and maintaining the T, kick your left foot out to the side.

3 Dismount by stepping off the dome with your left foot and lowering your arms.

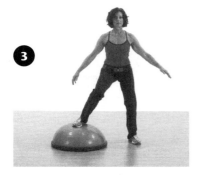

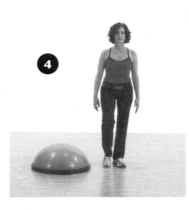

4 Tap your right foot lightly beside your left foot.

Repeat 4–5 times, then start over on the other side.

TIPS

- Stay erect. Avoid leaning to the side as you kick.
- Contract your core, especially your lower abs, to stabilize.

Count	1	2	3	4
Cue	Step	Kick	Step	Tap

STARTING POSITION: Stand on the dome with your feet about hip-width apart and your hips, knees, and toes facing forward. Raise your arms to the ceiling, keeping them straight and your palms facing forward.

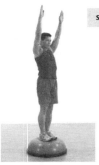

starting position

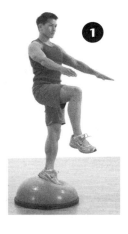

1

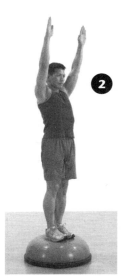

2

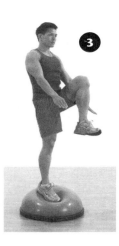

3

1 Bend and lift your right knee to around 90º. At the same time, arc your arms down until they're on either side of your knee. Your palms should face down.

2 Step down onto the dome with your right foot and arc your arms back up to the ceiling.

3 Repeat steps 1 and 2 on the other side, lifting your left knee.

Repeat 4–5 times.

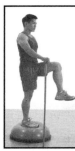

BASIC
Keep your hands in front of you and touch the palm of your hand to the knee that you lift. If you feel unsteady, hold a prop, like a body bar or broomstick, for balance.

Count	1	2	3	4
Cue	Step	Lift	Step	Lift

TIPS
- Stand firmly on the dome with your supporting leg.
- Engage your core vigorously to help you stabilize.
- Keep your knees slightly bent for stability.

STARTING POSITION: Stand a comfortable distance behind the dome with your feet about hip-width apart. Rest your hands by your sides.

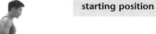
starting position

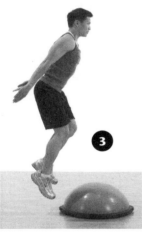

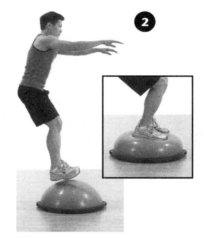

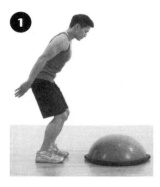

1 Bend your knees to prepare. Focus on the bull's eye. At the same time, swing your arms backward.

2 Jump with both feet onto the dome, swinging your arms forward. Exhale as you land firmly on bent knees, with your feet on either side of the bull's eye and your knees over your toes.

3 Dismount by jumping back to the floor with both feet.

Repeat 4–5 times.

BASIC
Instead of jumping off, dismount by stepping off the dome one foot at a time.

CHALLENGE
Move to the left side of the dome and try the same two-foot jump from the side to the top of the dome. Dismount by jumping down to the side, landing on both feet.

SUPER CHALLENGE
Combine forward and side jumps randomly. Do the jumps as continuously as possible.

TIPS
• Engage your core and stay connected from head to toe.

STARTING POSITION: Stand on the dome with your feet about hip-width apart and your hips, knees, and toes facing forward. Rest your hands by your sides.

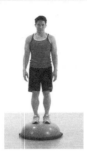

starting position

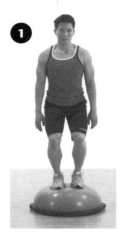

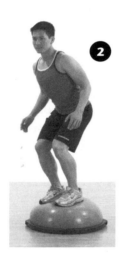

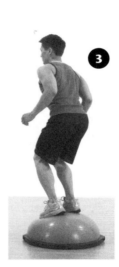

1–2 Bend your knees to prepare, then jump to face your right corner, landing firmly on bent knees.

3 Continue jumping in one direction eight times until you return to the front.

Start over on the other side. Then alternate directions.

Repeat 4–5 times.

BASIC
Jump to your right corner (eighth turn), then jump back to center. Now jump to your left corner, then jump back to center.

CHALLENGE
Instead of eighth turns, go around the dome in quarter-turn jumps.

SUPER CHALLENGE
Try half-turn jumps around the dome.

TIPS
- "Spot" your turn: Pick a point to turn to and land with your eyes. Your feet will follow.
- Keep your core tight.

STARTING POSITION: Stand on the dome with your hips, knees, and toes facing forward. Roll your hands into fists in front of your body, as if you're holding ski poles.

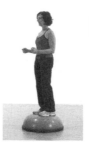

starting position

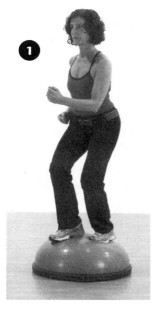

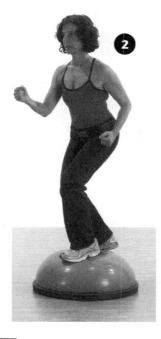

1 Bend your knees softly to prepare, then jump up slightly and land with your right foot forward and your left foot back. At the same time, move your arms in opposition to your feet.

2 Jump again and switch feet so that your left foot is forward and right foot is back. At the same time, move your arms in opposition to your feet.

Repeat several times, gradually adding speed.

CHALLENGE

Alternate between two single jumps (one jump on each side) and one double jump (two jumps on the same side), so the pattern is "single, single, double." Then try jumping a little higher on the second of the double jumps.

TIPS

- Face forward and look straight ahead.
- Stay low and move just your lower body
- Engage your core to keep your upper and lower body connected.

STARTING POSITION: Stand on the dome with your hips, knees, and toes facing forward. Roll your hands into fists in front of your body, as if you're holding ski poles.

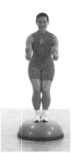

starting position

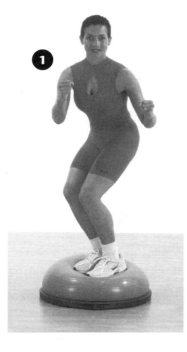

1

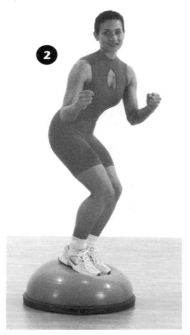

2

1 Bend your knees slightly to prepare, then jump to face your right corner by twisting from your hips but keeping your shoulders facing forward. Stay low and keep your knees and feet together.

2 Continuing to keep your shoulders facing forward, jump to face your left corner.

Repeat several times, gradually adding speed.

CHALLENGE

For fun, alternate between two single jumps (one jump on each side) and one double jump (two jumps on the same side), so the pattern is "single, single, double." Then try jumping a little higher on the second of the double jumps.

TIPS

- Face forward and look straight ahead.
- Keep your upper body still; move only your hips and legs.

STARTING POSITION: Stand on the dome with your feet about hip-width apart and your hips, knees, and toes facing forward. Roll your hands into fists in front of your body, as if you're holding ski poles.

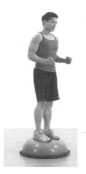

starting position

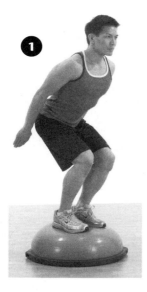

1

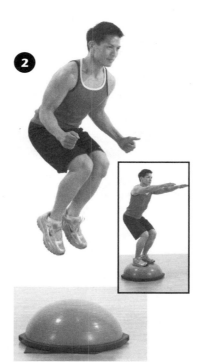

2

1 Bend your knees to prepare. At the same time, swing your arms behind you.

2 Jump up as high as you can with control. Land firmly on bent knees with your feet on either side of the bull's eye. At the same time, tuck your elbows into your body.

Repeat steps 1–2 several times, jumping a little higher each time until you can tuck your feet underneath you while you're in the air.

TIPS

- Brace yourself as you land and stay connected from head to toe.

squats and lunges

Squats and lunges target the glutes, hamstrings, and quads. They also challenge your core and help build stable knees, feet, and ankles. In addition, lunges tend to put the body off balance because of their wider stance. You need stable hips and shoulders to offset this inclination, and that means you need a very strong core, since the core muscles help stabilize the pelvis and spine.

When we squat or lunge on an unstable surface like the BOSU, there's the added dimension of balance to contend with—and this is no small feat! All told, squatting and lunging on the dome take strength, stability, and a very strong connection between your upper and lower body. The exercises in this section help you work toward that goal.

Helpful hints

- Connect to your core and brace yourself from your pelvic floor up to your shoulders.

- Keep your feet level on the dome. Avoid rolling them in or out.
- Make sure your hips are level and face forward.
- Keep your head in line with your spine.
- Keep your shoulders over your hips and your knees over your toes.
- When you lunge, plant your dome foot in the middle of the bull's eye and stand firmly on your supporting leg.

squat and over-the-top combo

STARTING POSITION: Stand a comfortable distance to the left of the dome with your feet about hip-width apart and your hips, knees, and toes facing forward. Rest your hands by your sides.

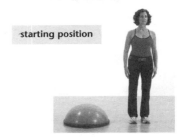

starting position

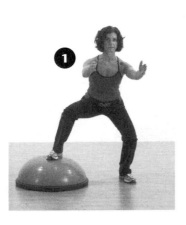

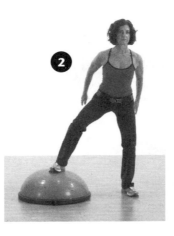

1 Step firmly onto the center of the dome with your right foot and bend both knees into a squat. At the same time, swing your arms forward.

2 Staying in your squat position, straighten up slightly and swing your arms back.

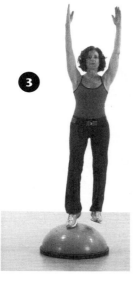

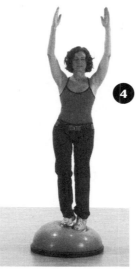

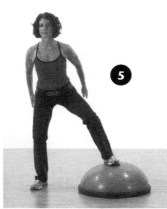

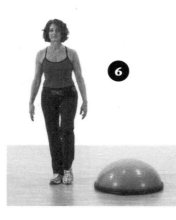

3 Transfer your weight to your right foot. At the same time, swing your arms overhead.

4 Keeping your arms overhead, step onto the dome with your left foot.

5 Dismount by stepping off the dome to the right with your right foot. At the same time, swing your arms back down to your sides.

6 Tap your left foot on the floor beside your right foot and swing your arms slightly backward.

Start over on the other side. Then alternate from side to side.

CHALLENGE

Speed up and add some bounce or propulsion to your steps. Spring off the first foot and replace it with the second foot as you go over the top of the BOSU.

SUPER CHALLENGE

Repeat the Challenge variation while holding a pair of hand weights.

Count	1	2	3	&	4	&
Cue	Down	Up	Over	The	Top	And

TIPS

- Keep your back straight.
- Push into your heels as you straighten up to activate your glutes and hamstrings.

STARTING POSITION: Stand on the dome with your feet about hip-width apart and your hips, knees, and toes facing forward. Rest your hands by your sides.

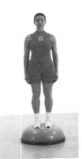

starting position

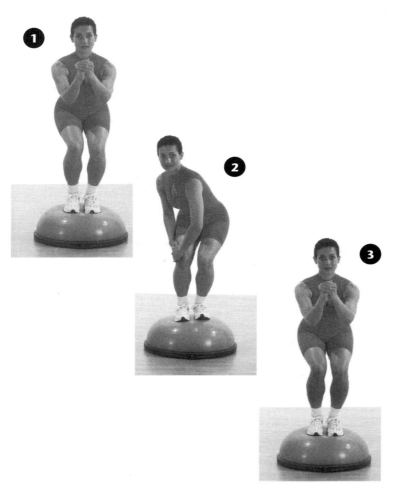

1 Squat down. At the same time, bend your arms and clasp your hands in front of you.

2 Keeping your hands clasped, twist from your waist to the right without moving your hips or knees. Touch the outside of your right knee.

3 Stay in your squat and twist back to center.

Count	1	2	3	4	5	6	7	8
Cue		Squat down		Twist	Center	Twist	Center	Straighten up

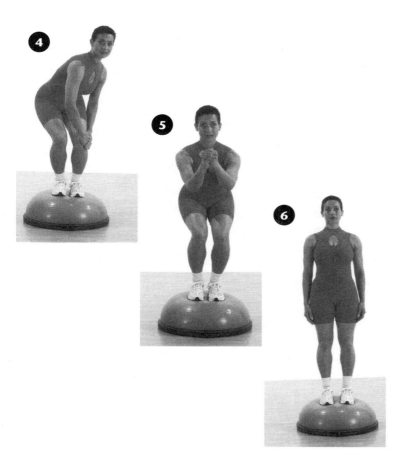

4 Maintaining your squat, twist to the left and touch the outside of your left knee.

5 Twist back to center.

6 Straighten up to your starting position.

Repeat 4–5 times.

CHALLENGE

For a visual challenge, follow your arms with your eyes as you twist.

SUPER CHALLENGE

Hold a weighted ball in front of your torso and deepen your squat as you do the exercise. Notice the increased demands on your core.

TIPS

• Engage your core vigorously to help you stabilize.

STARTING POSITION: Stand on the dome with your feet about hip-width apart and your hips, knees, and toes facing forward. Rest your hands by your sides.

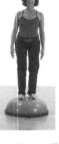
starting position

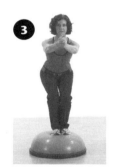

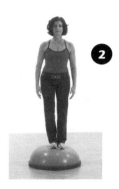

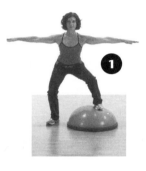

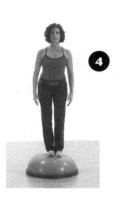

1 Step off the dome to your right with your right foot and land in a squat (the emphasis is down). At the same time, extend your arms to a T.

2 Straighten up and return your right foot to the top of the dome (the emphasis is up). Return your hands to your sides.

3 Squat down on top of the dome (the emphasis is down). At the same time, clasp your hands in front of you.

4 Straighten up to your starting position (the emphasis is up).

Start over on the other side. Then alternate from side to side.

Repeat 4–5 times.

Count	1	2	3	4
Cue	Squat	Up	Squat	Up

TIPS

- Stay centered over your hips as you move.
- Keep your knees over your toes throughout, especially as you squat.

STARTING POSITION: Stand on the dome with your feet about hip-width apart and your hips, knees, and toes facing forward. Rest your hands by your sides.

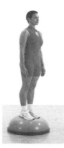

starting position

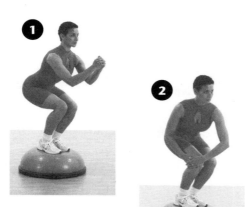

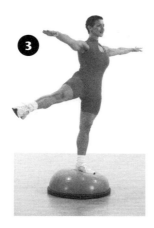

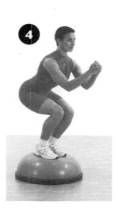

1 Engage your lower abs and squat down. At the same time, bend your arms and clasp your hands in front of you.

2 Keeping your hands clasped, twist from your waist to the right without moving your hips or knees. Touch the side of your right knee.

3 Twist back to center and lift your right leg as you straighten up. At the same time, arc your arms down and then extend them out to a T.

4 Lower you arms and leg and move straight into a squat as you start over on the other side.

Alternate from side to side.

Repeat 4–5 times.

Count	1	2	3	4
Cue	Squat	Twist	Lift	Down

TIPS

• Engage your inner thighs and core for stability.

STARTING POSITION: Stand on the dome with your feet about hip-width apart and your hips, knees, and toes facing forward. Roll your hands into fists in front of your body, as if you're holding ski poles.

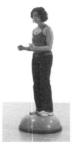

starting position

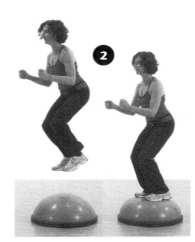

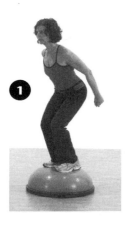

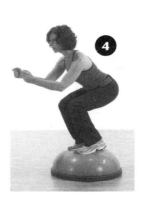

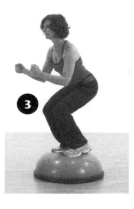

1 Bend your knees to prepare. As you bend, swing your arms back.

2 Jump up with both feet and land in a high squat, landing firmly with bent knees. Swing your arms forward as you land.

3 Repeat steps 1–2 but land in a medium, or deeper, squat.

4 Repeat steps 1–2 again, but land in a very deep squat.

Repeat 4–5 times.

TIPS
• Engage your inner thighs to help you stabilize.

STARTING POSITION: Stand a comfortable distance to the left of the dome with your feet together. Roll your hands into fists in front of your body.

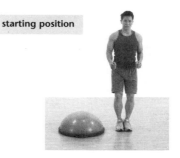

starting position

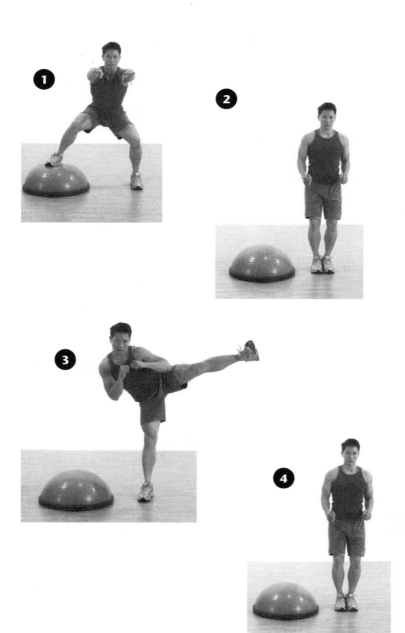

1 Step your right foot onto the dome and move into a squat. At the same time, arc your arms to shoulder height in front of you.

2 Step back to your starting position.

3 Transfer your weight to your right foot and kick your left foot out to your left side in kickboxing style. At the same time, bring your hands into your chest.

4 Lower your left foot back to its starting position.

Repeat 4–5 times, then start over on the other side.

TIPS

• Stand firmly on your supporting leg when you kick.
• Make sure the knee and foot of your kicking leg face forward.
• Keep your arms and shoulders braced throughout.

STARTING POSITION: Stand on the dome with your knees bent and your feet about hip-width apart. Rest your hands by your sides.

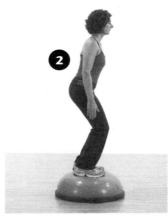

starting position

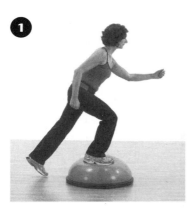

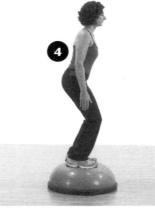

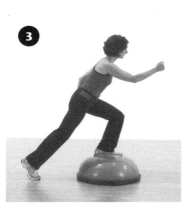

1 Transfer your weight onto your right foot and bend your right knee more. Now extend your left leg back until your toes touch the floor. At the same time, swing your left arm forward and your right arm back.

2 Step back onto the dome with your left foot.

3 Extend your right leg back until your toes touch the floor. At the same time, swing your right arm forward and your left arm back.

4 Step back onto the dome with your right foot and continue lunging from one foot to the other, gradually increasing speed.

Repeat several times.

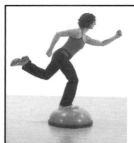

SUPER CHALLENGE

As you lunge, try extending your back foot in the air instead of touching your toes on the floor behind you.

TIPS

- Keep your knees over your toes.
- Lift your upper body out of your hips to stay forward and centered.
- Engage your core vigorously to offset the dome's rebound.

side lunge

STARTING POSITION: Stand on the dome with your knees bent and your feet about hip-width apart. Rest your hands by your sides.

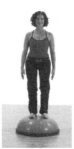

starting position

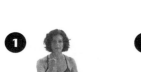

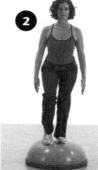

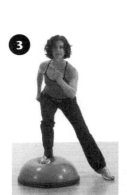

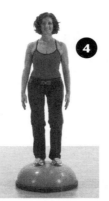

1 Transfer your weight onto your left foot and bend your left knee more. Now touch your right toe on the floor to the right of the dome. At the same time, swing your right arm in front of your torso.

2 Step back on the dome with your right foot.

3 Touch your left toe on the floor to the left of the dome. At the same time, swing your left arm in front of your torso.

4 Step back onto the dome with your left foot and continue lunging from side to side, gradually increasing speed.

Repeat several times.

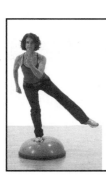

SUPER CHALLENGE
As you lunge, extend your active foot in the air instead of touching the dome or floor with your toe. Do one "air" lunge to each side and then hold the third one with your leg extended for an extra count.

TIPS
- Face forward and look straight ahead.
- Keep your knees over your toes.
- Engage your core to avoid leaning to the side and to offset the rebound from the dome.

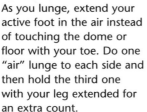
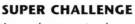

STARTING POSITION: Stand far enough behind the dome so that you can lunge forward and land on the bull's eye. Roll your hands into fists in front of your body.

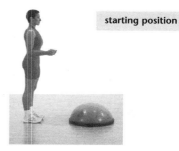

starting position

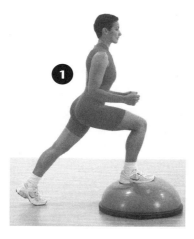

1

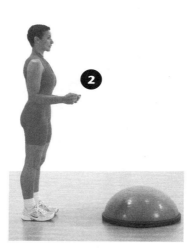

2

1 Lunge forward onto the dome with your right foot, aiming for the bull's eye. Land firmly with your supporting knee at right angles.

2 Step back to your starting position.

Alternate sides, this time lunging with your left foot. Repeat 5–10 times.

CHALLENGE
Bend and straighten your back leg while in the lunge position. Make sure both knees are bent at right angles.

SUPER CHALLENGE
Instead of lunging forward onto the dome and then stepping back, simultaneously exchange your feet from back to front and vice versa. Keep your weight forward as you exchange your feet.

TIPS
- Engage your core, especially your abs, to avoid arching your back.
- Make sure your hips are square and face forward.

STARTING POSITION: Stand far enough behind the dome so that you can lunge forward and land on the bull's eye. Roll your hands into fists in front of your body.

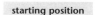
starting position

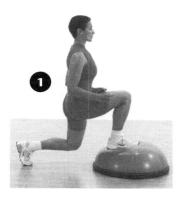

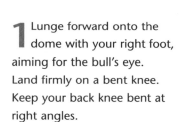

1 Lunge forward onto the dome with your right foot, aiming for the bull's eye. Land firmly on a bent knee. Keep your back knee bent at right angles.

2 Lift your right foot and stride back to a back lunge. Land with your right foot bent at right angles.

3 Lunge forward again, then continue to lunge back and forth.

Repeat 4–5 times, then start over on the other side.

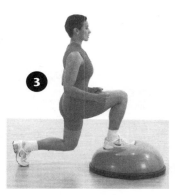

CHALLENGE
Do this exercise holding a free weight in each hand.

TIPS
- Engage your core, especially your abs, to avoid arching your back.
- Keep your torso upright and make sure your hips are square and facing forward.

abs and core

The exercises in this section target the deeper abdominals—the obliques and transversus abdominis—and other core muscles. Core muscles stabilize your spine, pelvis, and shoulders and provide a foundation of strength by transforming the abdomen and spine into a rigid cylinder. The stronger your core, the more stable and connected you are and the more skillfully and effectively you can move.

As you work through the exercises in this section, pull in your corset, squeeze the sponge in your belly, pull up your zipper muscles, or draw your belly button toward your spine—whatever image works—to help you engage and strengthen the pelvic floor and deep abdominals. In addition to strengthening specific muscle groups, the exercises in this section train you to use your body as a unit. Doing so on an unstable surface adds significant challenge. It also fine-tunes the nervous system to work better—on the BOSU and off.

Note: Many of these exercises require you to find your center of gravity on the dome.

For more information, see page 42.

Helpful hints

- Take the time to set up properly. Good alignment is half the battle.
- Center yourself and distribute your weight evenly.
- Connect to your core. Brace yourself from your pelvic floor up to your shoulders.
- Exhale audibly through your mouth on exertion to connect to your abs, especially your obliques.

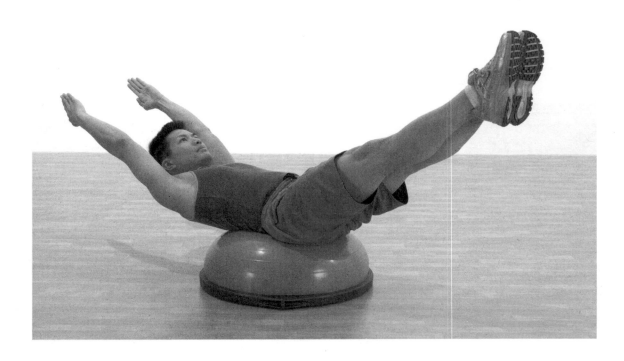

ab curl

STARTING POSITION: Lie face-up with your lower back on top of the dome and your upper body fully extended over the dome. Bend your knees and place your feet about hip-width apart on the floor. Keep your head in line with your spine and clasp your hands behind your head.

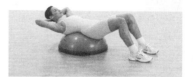

starting position

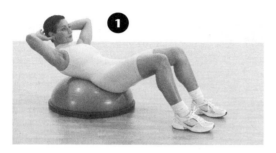

1

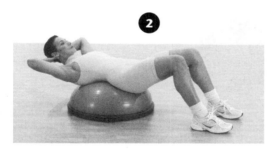

2

1 Slightly nod your head toward your chest and curl your upper body forward. Keep the back of your neck long and curl forward from your ribs as far as you can.

2 Slowly roll back through each vertebra to your starting position.

Repeat 5–10 times.

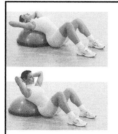

BASIC

Sit on the floor in front of the dome with your knees bent and feet flat on the floor. Let your upper back, shoulders, and head rest on the dome and clasp your hands behind your head. Curl forward as far as you can, then roll back down to your starting position.

CHALLENGE

Reach your left leg out in front of you as you extend your upper body backwards. Then bend your knee and fold your leg in toward your chest as you curl forward. Curl as far forward as possible.

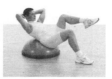

TIPS

• Engage your core, especially your lower abs, to help keep your hips level.

STARTING POSITION: Lie face-up with your lower back on the dome. Bend your knees 90º and keep your feet in line with your knees. Clasp your hands behind your head and keep your head in line with your spine. *Note:* Adjust your position as necessary to find your center of gravity.

starting position

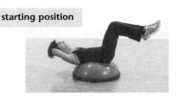

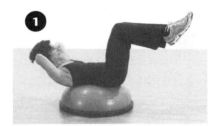

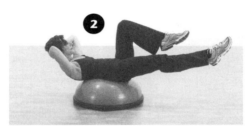

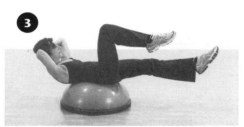

1 Slightly nod your head in toward your chest and curl your upper body forward. Keep the back of your neck long and curl forward from your ribs as far as you can.

2 Maintaining your curl, extend your right leg straight out in front of you to eye level. At the same time, bend your left leg in toward your chest.

3 Still in your curl, switch your legs so that your left leg is extended and your right leg is bent.

Repeat 5–10 times.

BASIC
Raise your legs higher (e.g., to 45º) to take the pressure off your lower back.

TIPS
• Engage your core throughout, especially as you switch your legs back and forth.

STARTING POSITION: Lie face-up with your lower back on the dome. Bend your knees 90º and keep your feet in line with your knees. Clasp your hands behind your head and keep your head in line with your spine. *Note:* Adjust your position as necessary to find your center of gravity.

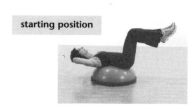

starting position

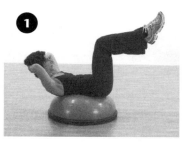

1 Slightly nod your head in toward your chest and curl your upper body forward. Keep the back of your neck long and curl forward from your ribs as far as you can.

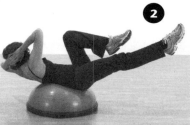

2 Maintaining your curl, extend your right leg straight out in front of you to eye level. At the same time, bend your left leg in toward your chest and twist your upper body toward your left knee.

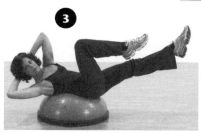

3 Still in your curl, switch your legs so that your left leg is extended and your right leg is bent. At the same time, twist your upper body toward your right knee.

Repeat 5–10 times.

SUPER CHALLENGE

Touch your elbow to the floor as you twist. For example, if you twist to the right, touch your right elbow to the floor beside the right side of the dome. (In this case, your left leg is extended and your right knee is bent.)

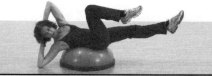

TIPS

- Stay out of your shoulders.
- Engage your core throughout, especially as you switch your legs back and forth.

STARTING POSITION: Lie face-up with your body fully extended on the dome. Stretch your arms back and straighten your legs, pointing your knees to the ceiling.

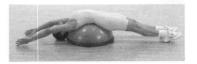

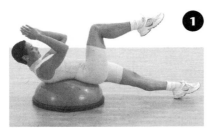

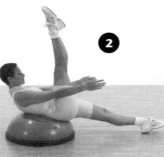

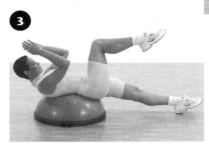

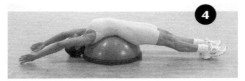

1 Bend your right knee in toward your chest. At the same time bend your elbows in toward your waist and start to curl your upper body forward.

2 Continue to curl your upper body forward and straighten your right leg toward the ceiling. At the same time, extend your arms forward on either side of your extended leg.

3 Start to uncurl your upper body. At the same time, bring your elbows back to your waist and bend your right leg toward your chest.

4 Stretch back to your starting position.

Start over on the other side. Then alternate from side to side.

Repeat 4–5 times.

BASIC
Hold the calf of your raised leg with both hands and, keeping that knee bent, climb up that leg as if it were a rope or a tree.

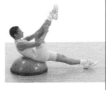

CHALLENGE
As you get more comfortable, speed up the sequence and make the movements smoother and even: Curl in, and up, uncurl, and lower back down.

TIPS
• Engage your core, especially your abs.

STARTING POSITION: Sit on the dome with your hips on or slightly in front of the bull's eye. Place your feet hip-width apart and flat on the floor. Lightly press your hands, either comfortably behind or beside you, into the dome. *Note:* Throughout this exercise, adjust your position as necessary to find your center of gravity.

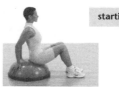

starting position

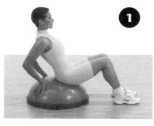

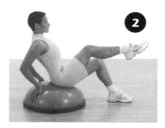

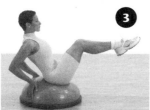

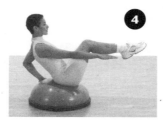

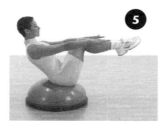

1 Engaging your lower abs vigorously to support your back, lean back slightly.

2 Holding your back steady, slowly bend and lift your right leg so that your right shin is parallel to the floor. Hold this position for 1 or 2 counts.

3 Slowly bend and lift your left leg so that your left shin is parallel to the floor. Hold both legs in the air for 1 or 2 counts.

4 Slowly lift your right arm until it's parallel to the floor and hold your arm and legs in the air for 1 or 2 counts.

5 Add your left arm, lifting it until it's parallel to the floor. Hold both arms and legs in the air for 1 or 2 counts.

Repeat 4–5 times.

TIPS

- Brace your shoulders and upper torso.
- Keep your head in line with your spine. Avoid dropping your chin or collapsing your chest.

SUPER CHALLENGE

Holding both legs up and extending both arms forward, extend your legs from your knees so that they're straight and you're in a full V-sit position.

STARTING POSITION: Sit on the dome with your hips on or slightly in front of the bull's eye. Place your feet hip-width apart and flat on the floor. Rest your hands by your sides. *Note:* Adjust your position as necessary to find your center of gravity.

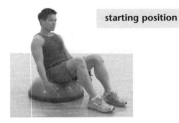
starting position

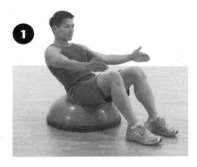
1

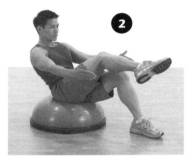
2

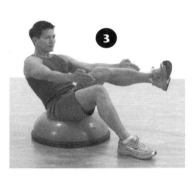
3

1 Engaging your lower abs vigorously, lean back slightly. At the same time, extend your arms in front of you.

2 Holding your back steady, slowly bend and lift your right leg. Without changing the shape of your leg, rotate it about 45° to the left.

3 Put your right foot down, then lift and rotate your left leg.

Repeat 4–5 times.

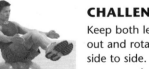

CHALLENGE
Keep both legs lifted throughout and rotate them from side to side. Then try moving your arms in opposition.

SUPER CHALLENGE
Keeping both legs lifted, hold a weighted ball in front of your torso and rotate from side to side. The added weight engages your core at a whole new level.

TIPS

• Keep your head in line with your spine. Avoid dropping your chin or collapsing your chest.

STARTING POSITION: Sit on the dome with your hips on or slightly in front of the bull's eye. Place your feet hip-width apart and flat on the floor. Lightly press your hands, comfortably behind you, into the dome. *Note:* Adjust your position as necessary to find your center of gravity.

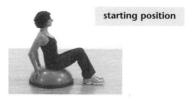

starting position

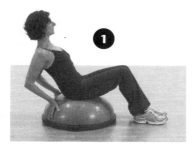

1 Engaging your lower abs vigorously, lean back slightly.

2 Bend your right knee in toward your chest. At the same time, straighten your left leg, keeping your heel on the floor.

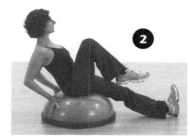

3 Switch legs so that your left leg is bent in toward your chest and your right leg is straight.

Repeat steps 2–3 several times.

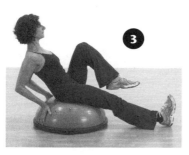

CHALLENGE

With your arms out in front, extend and lift your right leg to hip height as you bend your left leg in toward your chest. Then switch feet. Alternate back and forth several times with your feet in the air.

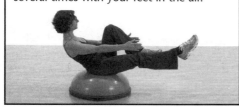

TIPS

- Draw in your low belly and pelvic floor to engage your core, especially your abs.

STARTING POSITION: Lie face-up with your lower back on the dome. Bend your knees 90º and keep your feet in line with your knees. Extend your arms forward and parallel to the floor. Keep your head in line with your spine. *Note:* Adjust your position as necessary to find your center of gravity.

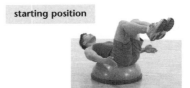
starting position

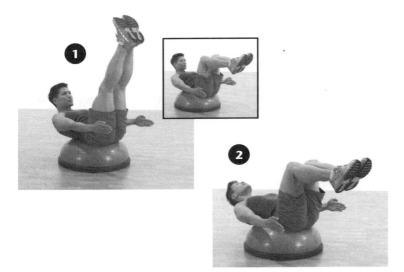

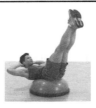

1 Slightly nod your head in toward your chest and curl your upper body forward. At the same time, extend your legs until your toes point to the ceiling.

2 Uncurl and return to your starting position.

Repeat 4–5 times.

BASIC
Try the exercise with your hands clasped behind your head. Curl your upper body forward and extend your legs toward the ceiling. Stay curled and raise and lower your legs from 90º.

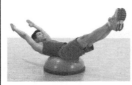

SUPER CHALLENGE
Move your arms and legs away from their vertical positions a little further each time you do the exercise. Ultimately, the goal is to extend your legs out at a 45º angle while your arms reach straight back beside your ears. This variation requires a very strong core so be careful and try it in stages.

TIPS
- Draw in your low belly and pelvic floor to engage your core, especially your abs.

STARTING POSITION: Sit with your hips centered on top of the dome. Extend your legs forward, keeping your feet flexed and your heels on the floor. Rest your arms along your sides, reaching your fingers toward your toes.

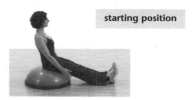

starting position

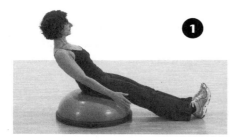

1 Contract your low belly and pelvic floor and lean straight back, hinging from your hips, until you feel some tension in your lower abs. Hold for 2 counts, then hinge back up to your starting position.

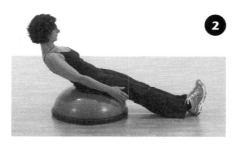

2 Repeat the exercise but lean back one more inch. Hold for 2 counts, then straighten up to your starting position.

3 This time, hold at the lowest point you can without arching or straining your back. Hold for 2 counts. Then straighten up to your starting position.

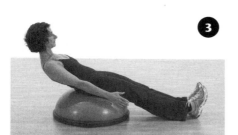

TIPS

- Keep your shoulders wide and your neck relaxed.
- Avoid arching your back and popping your rib cage forward.

STARTING POSITION: Lie face-up with your lower back on the dome and your torso extended back until it's parallel to the floor. Keep your legs together with your knees bent and feet flat on the floor. Hold your arms by your sides and keep your head in line with your spine. *Note:* Adjust your position as necessary to find your center of gravity.

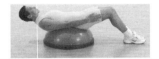

starting position

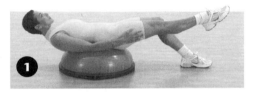

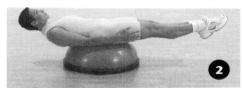

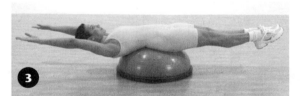

1 Engaging your core, especially your lower abs, extend your right leg straight out in front of you until it's the same height as your left knee.

2 Extend your left leg until it's the same height as your right leg.

3 Stretch your arms overhead behind you and try to get your body as parallel to the floor as possible. Hold for 5 counts. Then return to your starting position.

Repeat 4–5 times.

BASIC

Extend your right leg straight out in front of you until it's the same height as your left knee. At the same time, extend your arms overhead behind you. Lower your leg and repeat with your left leg extended.

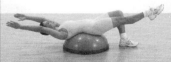

TIPS

• Keep your shoulders wide and your neck relaxed.

• Avoid arching your back and popping your rib cage forward.

Caution: Avoid this exercise if you have wrist problems.

STARTING POSITION: Assume a full plank position: Your feet are flexed and your toes are centered on top of the dome. Your hands are on the floor directly under your shoulders. Your arms are straight. Your body is in a straight line from head to foot.

starting position

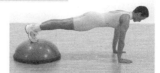

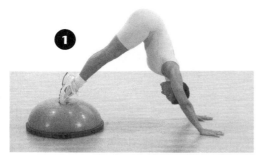

1 Press down into your hands and draw in your abs to lift your hips up until your body forms an inverted V and you are on the tips of your toes.

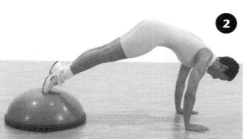

2 Slowly lower back out to your plank position.

Repeat 4–5 times.

BASIC

Lie face-down with your shins, knees, and lower thighs on the dome. Clasp your hands and form a triangle on the floor with your elbows and hands. Contract your abs and slowly pull your thighs toward your head to pike your hips up a little bit.

SUPER CHALLENGE

Simultaneously lift one leg while piking to your inverted V. Avoid rotating your hip out as you lift your leg.

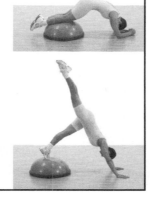

TIPS

• Draw in your low belly and pelvic floor to keep from sagging and arching your back.

back and bridge exercises

Back exercises are particularly important because we live most of our lives facing and bending forward. We rarely do the reverse. Yet we need strong backs for support. The exercises in this section focus on the back but work the whole body. The first set of exercises targets the middle and upper back muscles. The remaining exercises are executed in a bridge position.

Working in a bridge position targets the glutes and hamstrings and helps to open the hip flexors and quads at the front of our hips and legs. These muscles are often short-ened by all the bending and sitting we do. Bridge exercises also demand a strong core to keep the pelvis and shoulders stable, and active adductors to keep our knees in line with our feet.

Note: Some of these exercises require you to find your center of gravity on the dome. For more information, see page 25.

Helpful hints

- Engage your obliques and lower abs to support your back.

When executing back exercises:
- Keep your neck long, your head in line with your spine, and your shoulders away from your ears.
- Extend through the front of your hips and keep your legs straight.

When you're in bridge position:
- Keep your feet parallel and in line with your hips and knees.
- Activate your adductors, hamstrings, and glutes to prevent your knees from splaying open.
- Distribute your weight evenly between your feet and across your shoulders. Don't arch your back.

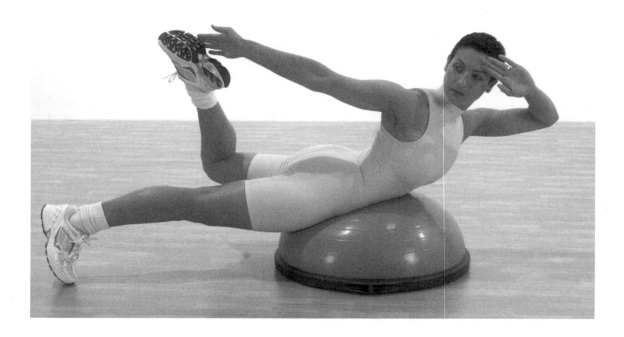

STARTING POSITION: Lie face-down with your abdomen centered on the dome. Rest your arms on the floor in front of you and extend your legs behind you. Keep your head in line with your spine. *Note:* Adjust your position as necessary to find your center of gravity.

starting position

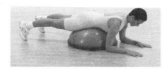

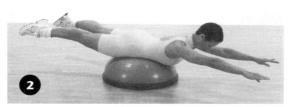

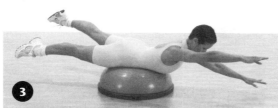

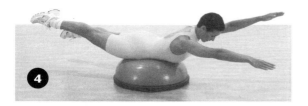

1 Slowly extend and lift both legs slightly off the floor. Lift your legs from your glutes and keep your legs very straight.

2 Slowly extend and lift both arms slightly off the floor.

3 Staying in this extended position, slowly raise your right arm and left leg higher than the left arm and right leg. Hold for 1 count.

4 Lower your right arm and left leg and raise your left arm and right leg higher. Hold for 1 count.

Repeat steps 3–4 several times, gradually adding speed.

BASIC

Slowly lift and lower one leg at a time off the floor. Then slowly lift and hold one arm at a time. Next, lift both arms at the same time. Finally lift both legs at the same time.

TIPS

- Engage your core, especially your abs, to avoid arching your back and popping your rib cage forward.

STARTING POSITION: Lie face-down with your abdomen centered on the dome. Rest your arms on the floor in front of you. Keep your head in line with your spine. *Note:* Adjust your position as necessary to find your center of gravity.

starting position

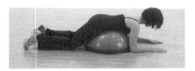

1 Draw in your low belly, then slowly lift and extend both arms in a V in front of you. Keep your arms slightly bent and your neck long.

2 Slowly lift and extend both legs behind you, allowing your legs to be slightly bent. Hold for 5 counts.

3 Slowly lower your arms and legs with control.

Repeat 4–5 times.

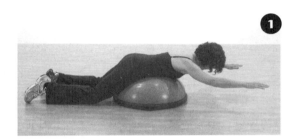

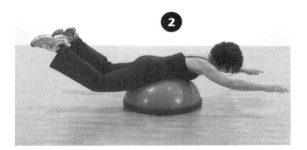

BASIC
Do the exercise without lifting your arms off the floor.

SUPER CHALLENGE
With arms and legs extended, tilt your body to one side, then to the center, then to the other side. For more challenge, add a straight-leg flutter kick as you tilt.

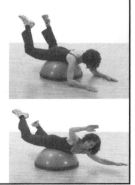

TIPS
- Relax your shoulders. Keep them away from your ears!
- Engage your core, especially your abs, to support your back.

STARTING POSITION: Lie face-down with your pelvis and lower abdomen centered on the dome. Extend your legs straight behind you and flex your feet, keeping your toes on the floor. Bend your elbows and place your palms on the floor. Rest your forehead on the backs of your hands. *Note:* Adjust your position as necessary to find your center of gravity.

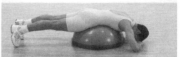

starting position

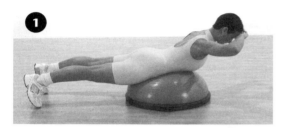

1 Draw in your low belly then slowly move into a back extension by peeling your upper body off the dome. Lift as far as you can without straining or crunching the back of your neck. Hold for 1 count.

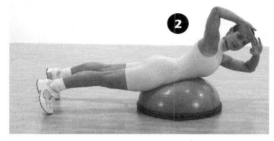

2 At the top, twist from your waist to your right.

3 Twist back to center.

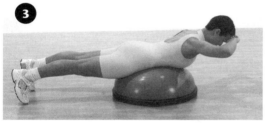

4 Slowly lower your upper body and return to your starting position.

Start over and twist to the other side.

Repeat 4–5 times.

CHALLENGE

Extend and lift your left leg as you move into a back extension and twist to the right.

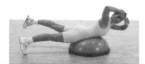

SUPER CHALLENGE

As you twist to the right side, extend your right arm out and behind you. Bend your left foot in and touch it with your right hand.

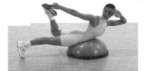

TIPS

- Press your hips evenly into the dome.
- Keep the backs of your hands glued to your forehead throughout the exercise.
- Engage your core, especially your lower abs, to protect your back and avoid over-arching.

STARTING POSITION: Lie face-down with your hips centered on top of the dome. Extend your legs straight behind you and flex your feet, keeping your toes on the floor. Rest your elbows and forearms on the floor in front of you.

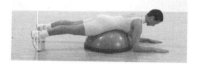

starting position

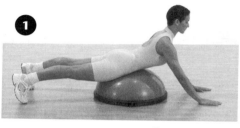

1

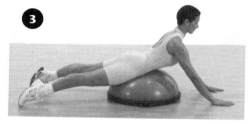

2

3

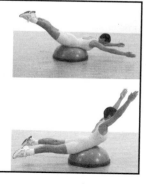

1 Draw in your low belly and press into your hands to straighten up to a back extension. Hold for 2 counts.

2 Bend your elbows to lower your upper body. At the same time, keep your abs tight and extend and lift your legs straight out behind you.

3 Press back up to your extension and lower your legs back to the floor.

Repeat steps 2–3 another 4–5 times, using your abs to rock back and forth. As you lower your upper body, your legs lift. As you extend your upper body, your legs drop.

SUPER CHALLENGE

Do the exercise without arm support: Slide your arms off the floor straight in front of you. Use your abs (not momentum!) to rock back and forth so that your hands and feet alternately move up and down.

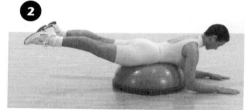

TIPS

- Keep your body taut throughout the exercise.
- Engage your core vigorously, especially your abs, to stay connected and move your body as a unit.

leg push

STARTING POSITION: Lie face-down with your torso bent over the dome. Rest your elbows and forearms on the floor in front of you.

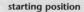
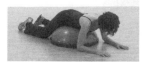
starting position

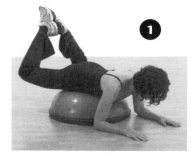

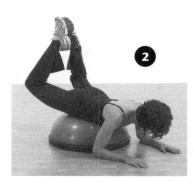

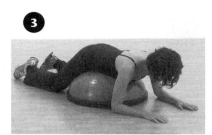

1 With your heels together, bend your knees and make a diamond shape with your legs.

2 Without changing the angle of your legs, push both feet up toward the ceiling from your glutes. Squeeze your feet together and keep your knees lifted. Hold for 2 counts.

3 Lower your legs to their starting position.

Repeat 4–5 times.

TIPS

- Contract your abs vigorously to avoid straining or arching your lower back.
- Squeeze your buttocks to engage your glutes and hamstrings.

STARTING POSITION: Lie on your back and place your feet about hip-width apart on top of the platform. Rest your hands by your sides.

starting position

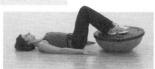

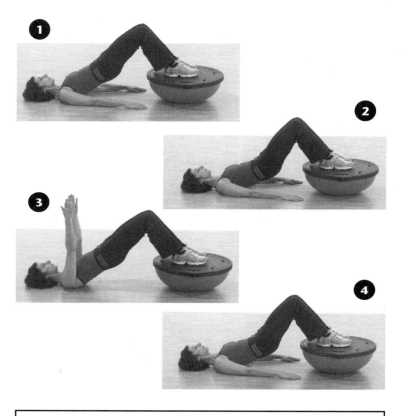

1 Press into your feet and slowly roll your hips up off the floor until you're in a bridge position. Keep your back ribs in contact with the floor.

2 Slowly roll back to your starting position one vertebra at a time. Then repeat steps 1–2 a few more times.

3 Extend your arms to the ceiling then press up to a bridge position.

4 Slowly roll back to your starting position one vertebra at a time. Then repeat steps 3–4 a few more times.

CHALLENGE

From your bridge position, press your feet into the platform to tilt it to the right, to the center, to the left, and to the center again. Then tilt it forward, to the center, backward, and to the center again.

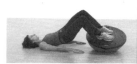

SUPER CHALLENGE

Bend and lift one leg off the platform slightly and place your supporting foot in the middle of the platform. Slowly roll your hips up to a bridge position on your supporting leg. Then roll your hips back down and repeat on the other side.

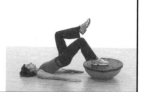

TIPS

- Keep your knees in line with your toes throughout.
- Continue to press into your feet to keep your hips lifted.
- Lift from your hamstrings and glutes, not from your back.

STARTING POSITION: Place yourself in a bridge position so that the midline of your body is about 12 inches to the left of the bull's eye. The right side of your body rests on the dome; the left side is off the dome. Keep your hips lifted, knees bent, and feet flat on the floor. Reach your arms out to the sides in a T with your palms facing up.

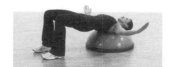

starting position

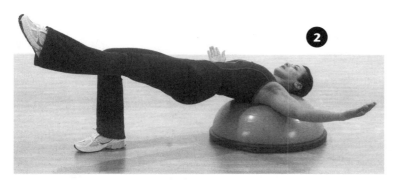

1 Press down on your left shoulder. At the same time, stand firmly on your right foot to keep your left hip level with your right hip.

2 Lift and extend your left leg to the height of your right knee. Hold for 5 counts. Then lower your leg to its starting position.

Repeat 4–5 times, then start over on the other side.

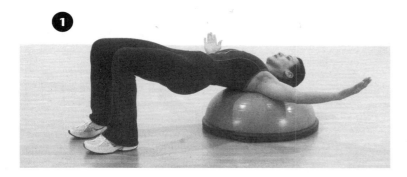

TIPS

• Draw in your low belly and pelvic floor to engage your core.

STARTING POSITION: Sit on the floor in front of the dome. Bend your knees and place your feet flat on the floor. Rest your upper back, shoulders, and head on the dome and clasp your hands behind your head.

starting position

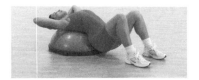

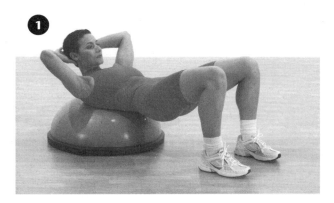

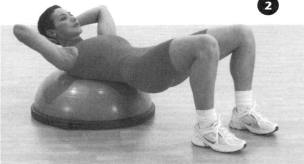

1 Press into your feet and roll your hips up to a bridge position. At the same time, curl your upper body forward into an ab curl.

2 Uncurl and roll back down one vertebra at a time.

Repeat 4–5 times.

CHALLENGE

Place your lower back on the dome and extend your upper body back from there. Do the ab curl and hip roll combination in this position.

SUPER CHALLENGE

With your upper back extended over the dome, lift one foot off the floor slightly. Do a one-legged hip roll and ab curl at the same time in this position.

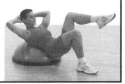

TIPS

• Press down into your feet, especially your heels, to activate your hamstrings and glutes.

• Keep the back of your neck long. Curl forward from your ribs.

plank, push-up, and side exercises

The exercises in this section all focus on the upper body, but rely extensively on core and other supporting muscles. Plank and push-up exercises require a good deal of strength and control. Working on the BOSU's unstable surface adds to the difficulty. So start small and build up slowly.

Side exercises target the obliques in a big way. They also require support from your glutes and core to stabilize the shoulders and pelvis and help you stay on your side. So once again, while the focus is a specific area, the entire body has to work to help you perform successfully.

Note: Avoid these exercises if you have wrist problems. Also, some of these exercises require you to find your center of gravity on the dome. For more information, see page 25.

Helpful hints

For plank and push-up exercises:
- Connect to your core and brace yourself from your pelvic floor up to your shoulders.
- Place your hands directly under your shoulders and avoid locking your elbows.

Elbow creases should face each other.
- Press into the heels of your hands to stay lifted through your shoulders.
- Keep your head in line with your spine.
- Avoid collapsing in the middle.

For side exercises:
- Engage your obliques and lower abs to keep your top hip from rolling backward.
- Keep your shoulders and hips stacked on top of each other (imagine lying between two panes of glass).

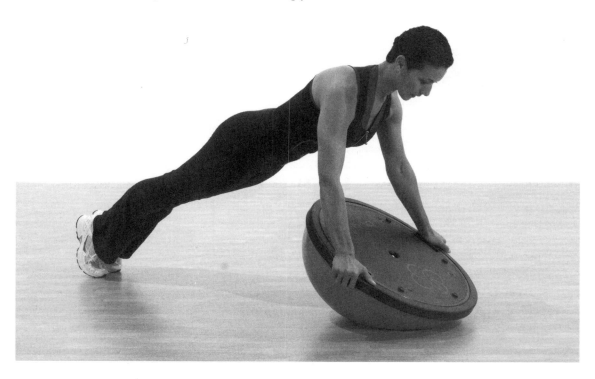

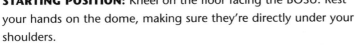

STARTING POSITION: Kneel on the floor facing the BOSU. Rest your hands on the dome, making sure they're directly under your shoulders.

starting position

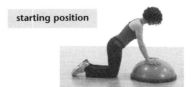

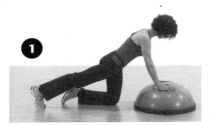

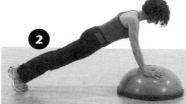

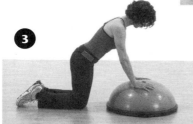

1 Contract your abs and extend your right leg straight back with your foot flexed on the floor. Keep your neck long and your head in line with your spine.

2 Extend your left leg back until you're in a full plank position. Press firmly into the heels of your hands to keep from sinking between your shoulder blades. Hold for 5 counts.

3 Return to your starting position one leg at a time.

Repeat 4–5 times.

BASIC

From your starting position, place your elbows on the dome. Clasp your hands and form a triangle with your elbows. Then extend your legs into an elbow plank position.

CHALLENGE

From a full plank position, lift and extend your right leg. Hold for 2 counts.

SUPER CHALLENGE

Take your extended leg out to the side. Go as far as you can without shifting your hips. Hold for 2 counts.

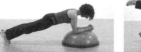

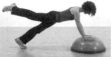

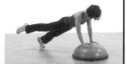

TIPS

- Keep your elbows soft. Avoid locking them to stay out of your neck muscles.
- Engage your lower abs to keep from straining your lower back.

platform plank

STARTING POSITION: Kneel on the floor facing the BOSU. Hold the handles on either side of the platform.

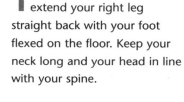

starting position

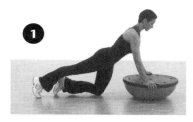

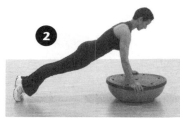

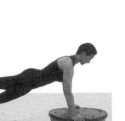

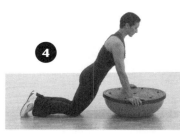

1 Contract your abs and extend your right leg straight back with your foot flexed on the floor. Keep your neck long and your head in line with your spine.

2 Extend your left leg back until you're in a full plank position. Press firmly into the heels of your hands to keep from sinking between your shoulder blades. Hold for 5 counts.

3 Lift and extend your right leg. Hold for 2 counts.

4 Return to your starting position one leg at a time.

Repeat 4–5 times.

BASIC
Do a basic plank position without lifting your leg.

CHALLENGE
From a full plank, lift and extend your right leg. Take that leg out to the side. Go only as far as you can without shifting your hips. Hold for 2 counts.

SUPER CHALLENGE
In your full plank position, tilt the BOSU forward, center, backward, and center. Then tilt it to the right, center, left, and center. When you're comfortable, make a continuous circle in one direction and then the other. *Caution:* Avoid this variation if you have wrist problems.

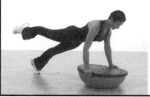

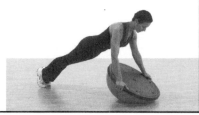

TIPS
- Keep your elbows soft. Avoid locking them to stay out of your neck muscles.
- Engage your lower abs to keep from straining your lower back.

STARTING POSITION: Hold the handles on either side of the platform and assume a full plank position.

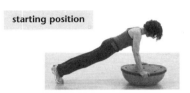

starting position

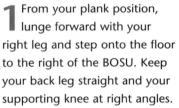

1 From your plank position, lunge forward with your right leg and step onto the floor to the right of the BOSU. Keep your back leg straight and your supporting knee at right angles.

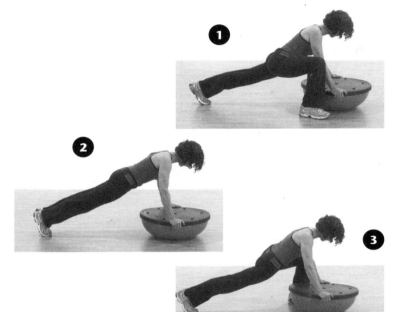

2 Return to your starting plank position.

3 Lunge forward with your left leg and step onto the floor to the left of the BOSU.

4 Return to your plank position.

Repeat 5–10 times.

TIPS

- To help you move forward from the plank position, lift your hips up as you lunge forward.
- Draw in your low belly and pelvic floor to avoid sinking in your hips.
- Use your chest, upper back, and arm muscles to keep the BOSU level.

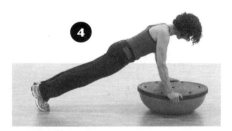

SUPER CHALLENGE

Speed up the lunges so that you're almost running in and out, alternating your feet simultaneously. Place your front foot just behind the dome instead of to the side.

dome push-up

STARTING POSITION: Place your hands on the sides of the dome and assume a full plank position.

starting position

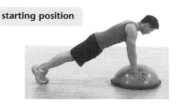

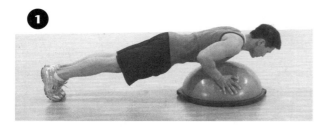

1

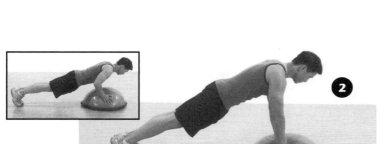

2

1 Bend your arms and lower your body down as far as you can without collapsing. Maintain a straight line from head to foot.

2 Use your chest, upper back, and arm muscles to push back up to a full plank position. Exhale as you straighten your arms to deepen the connection to your core.

Repeat 4–5 times.

BASIC
Do the push-up with your knees on the floor.

CHALLENGE
Extend and lift your right leg a few inches as you execute the push-up. Keep your extended leg as straight as possible and engage your core vigorously to avoid sagging in the middle.

SUPER CHALLENGE
Repeat the exercise as a triceps push-up: Place your hands closer together on the dome. Make sure your elbows stay close to your torso and point back as you execute the push-up.

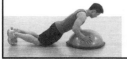

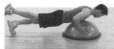

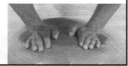

TIPS
- Engage your core, especially your abs, to keep your body taut and your hips from sinking.
- Press firmly from the heels of your hands to keep from sinking between your shoulder blades.

STARTING POSITION: Hold the handles on either side of the platform and assume a full plank position.

starting position

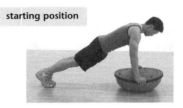

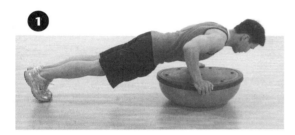

1 Bend your arms and lower your body down as far as you can without collapsing. Maintain a straight line from head to foot.

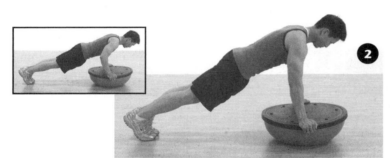

2 Use your chest, upper back, and arm muscles to push back up to a full plank position. Exhale as you straighten your arms to deepen the connection to your core.

Repeat 4–5 times.

BASIC
Do the push-up with your knees on the floor.

SUPER CHALLENGE
Extend and lift one leg a few inches while you execute the push-up. Keep your extended leg as straight as possible and engage your core vigorously to avoid sagging in the middle.

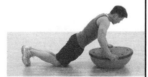

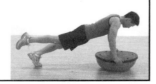

TIPS
- Engage your core, especially your abs, to keep your body taut and your hips from sinking.
- Press firmly from the heels of your hands to keep from sinking between your shoulder blades.

STARTING POSITION: Lie with your left hip on the dome, keeping your legs extended and your feet stacked on top of each other. Place your left forearm on the floor, with your left elbow directly under your shoulder, and rest your right hand in front of you on top of the dome. *Note:* Adjust your position as necessary to find your center of gravity.

starting position

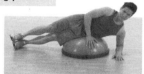

1

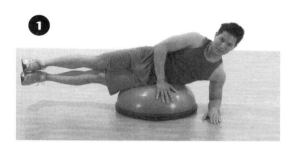

1 Using your right arm as a support, lift both legs off the floor to hip height.

2 Slowly lift your right arm off the dome and then lift your left arm off the floor. Cross both arms over your chest. Keep your body stiff and straight and make sure your head is in line with your spine. Hold for 5 counts.

2

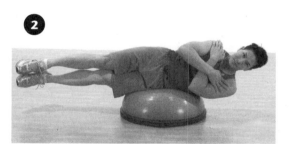

3 Release your arms and lower your legs.

Repeat 4–5 times, then start over on the other side.

3

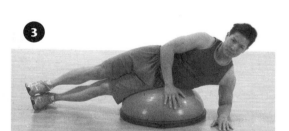

TIPS

• Engage your core, especially your abs and your inner thighs, to avoid arching your back or tucking your pelvis.

STARTING POSITION: Lie fully extended over the dome on your left hip and stack your hips on top of each other. Scissor your left leg forward and your right leg back, resting your feet on the floor. Extend your right arm overhead and support your head and neck with your left arm. *Note:* Adjust your position as necessary to find your center of gravity.

starting position

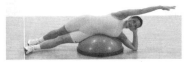

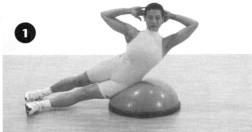

1 Engage your abs and curl up to the side, exhaling as you curl. At the same time, clasp both hands together behind your head.

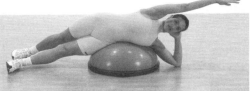

2 Lower your upper body, reaching your right arm back over your head again to stretch out your right side.

Repeat several times, then start over on the other side.

BASIC
Choose a wider scissor position for more stability.

CHALLENGE
As you curl up to the side, extend your upper arm straight out to the side so that it's parallel to the floor. At the same time, extend the bottom arm straight up to the ceiling.

SUPER CHALLENGE
Instead of doing the exercise in a stride stance, stack your feet on top of each other. Dig the side of your bottom foot into the floor, then place your other foot on top. Flex your feet.

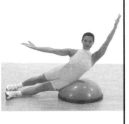

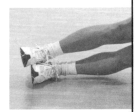

TIPS
• Keep your hips square and your body aligned from head to toe at all times.

STARTING POSITION: Lie with your right hip on the dome, keeping your hips stacked on top of each other. Extend your legs and let them hover above the floor. Place your right forearm on the floor, with your right elbow directly under your shoulder, and rest your left hand on your hip. *Note:* Adjust your position as necessary to find your center of gravity.

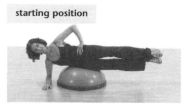

starting position

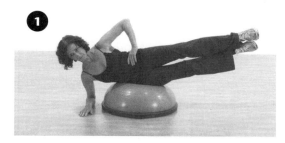

1 Keeping your legs in line with your body, lift both legs a few inches. Hold for 2 counts.

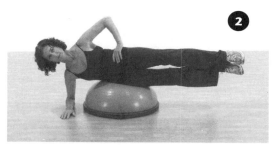

2 Lower your legs to their starting position.

Repeat 4–5 times, then start over on the other side.

BASIC
Lift only the top leg to hip height and then return to your starting position.

CHALLENGE
Lift the top leg a few inches. Then lift the bottom leg to meet it. Hold for 2 counts. Lower both legs to their starting position.

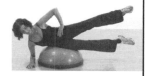

SUPER CHALLENGE
Curl your upper body up to the side and reach your top arm toward your feet as you lift both legs together.

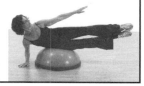

TIPS
- Engage your core, especially your abs, to help you stabilize your pelvis and avoid collapsing in your hips.
- Keep your legs in line with your body.

STARTING POSITION: Sit on the floor a comfortable distance to the left of the dome so that your legs are loosely bent and your top foot is slightly forward. Place your right forearm across the top of the dome at right angles to your body and rest your left hand on your waist.

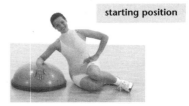
starting position

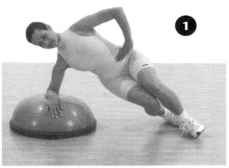
❶

1 Engage your abs and inner thighs and press into your right forearm to lift your right side off the floor. Exhale as you lift. Keep your neck long and your right shoulder over your elbow. Hold for 2 counts.

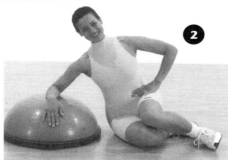
❷

2 Lower your hips to your starting position.

Repeat 4–5 times, then start over on the other side.

CHALLENGE

From your starting position, place your right hand on top of the dome. Press into your right hand and forward foot to lift your right side off the floor. Finish in a full side-plank position with straight arms and your legs and feet stacked on top of each other.

SUPER CHALLENGE

Raise the top leg while you're in the side plank.

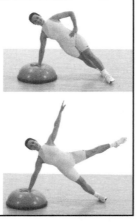

TIPS

• Keep your chest open and avoid sagging in the hip area.

kneeling and balance exercises

Kneeling plays with our balance because our brains and muscles have to adjust to a less familiar position and pattern of weight distribution. When we add the instability of the dome to the mix, there's a lot to contend with.

Balance also comes into play in countless daily activities. We balance when we stand on two feet, or on one foot to put on our shoes, or as we walk—perching on one foot until we overstep and our weight propels us to the other foot.

This all seems to come naturally. Yet when we deliberately try to balance, we often have trouble. Balancing requires a lot of systems working together—the eyes, ears, and other sensors, as well as the brain and the musculo-skeletal system. Success depends on many factors, including body alignment, the strength and tone of our muscles, and the amount of experience or "muscle memory" we have in each case.

The good news is that we can train ourselves to balance better. And the BOSU is an ideal tool to help. The exercises in this section focus on kneeling and other balancing positions as well as movements that challenge balance.

Helpful hints
- Practice on the floor first.
- Take your time to set up properly. Alignment is key in any balancing position.
- Focus on a point in front of you to help reduce the amount of visual information the brain has to process.
- Keep your shoulders and hips square.
- Connect to your core and brace yourself from your pelvic floor up to your shoulders.

For kneeling exercises:
- Avoid buckling at the hips.
- Squeeze your inner thighs together, engage your glutes, and press your shins into the dome to help you balance and stay erect.

For other balancing exercises:
- Consciously engage the hamstrings, adductors, and lower glutes of your supporting leg.

STARTING POSITION: Kneel upright on top of the dome, placing your right knee on the bull's eye and your left knee against the side of the dome. Hover your right toe off the floor behind you. Raise your arms out to the sides in a T.

starting position

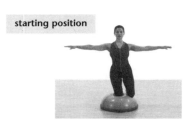

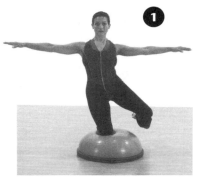

1 Without changing the shape and angle of your left leg, slowly lift your left knee to the side with control. Press your shin into the dome to help you stay erect. Hold for 2 counts.

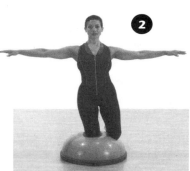

2 Lower the left knee back to the dome.

Repeat 4–5 times, then start over on the other side.

BASIC
Keep the toes of your supporting foot down to help you balance.

SUPER CHALLENGE
Raise your right knee, then take it around to the front, side, and back, holding for 2 counts in each position.

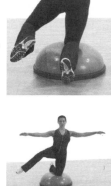

TIPS
- Contract your lower abs to keep your pelvis level, especially as you lift and lower your knee.
- Face forward and look straight ahead. Reach the crown of your head toward the ceiling.

STARTING POSITION: Kneel on top of the dome with your knees on either side of the bull's eye and your hands on top of the dome in front of you.

starting position

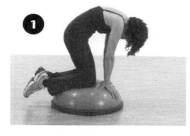

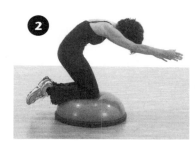

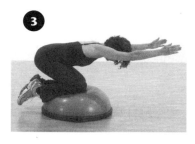

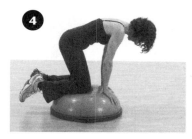

1 Press into your shins and round your back.

2 Lift and extend both arms out in front of you. Exhale to connect to your core and support your back.

3 Keep your arms extended and flatten to a straight back. Keep your upper body as parallel to the floor as possible.

4 Return to all fours.

Repeat 4–5 times.

BASIC
Keep your toes down to help you balance. Press into both hands and shins and round your back like an angry cat. Then lift and extend one arm at a time in front of your body.

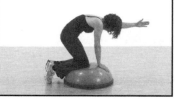

TIPS
• Engage your lower abs to help you tuck your pelvis under.

kneeling tracking drill

STARTING POSITION: Kneel upright on top of the dome with your knees on either side of the bull's eye. Hover your toes off the floor behind you. Extend your arms to the floor and point both hands to your right hip.

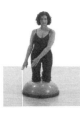

starting position

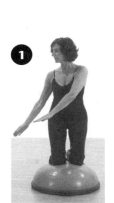

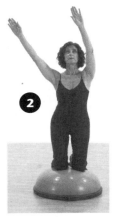

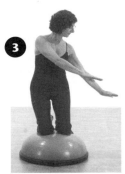

1 Lean slightly into your left hip but keep your hips square. At the same time, press into your shins and, moving both hands together, slowly arc your arms up to your right side.

2 Arc your arms over your head.

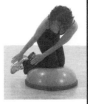

3 Then arc your arms down to your left hip. As you approach your left hip, lean slightly into your right hip.

4 Arc your arms back to their starting position.

Repeat 4–5 times, then start over on the other side.

BASIC
Do the exercise with your toes on the floor.

CHALLENGE
Touch your ankle, instead of your hip, as you rotate from side to side.

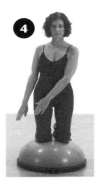

SUPER CHALLENGE
Trace a figure 8 in front of your torso, moving your hips from side to side in opposition to your arms. Follow your arm movements with your eyes.

TIPS
- Reach the crown of your head to the ceiling at all times.
- Keep your hips square to the front and press your shins into the dome.
- Engage your core muscles vigorously as you move your arms to prevent your hips from buckling.

STARTING POSITION: Kneel on top of the dome, placing your left knee on the bull's eye and extending your right leg straight out behind you with your toes touching the floor. Rest both hands on the floor in front of the dome.

starting position

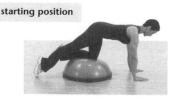

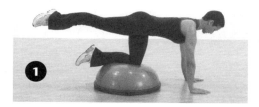

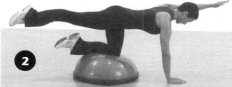

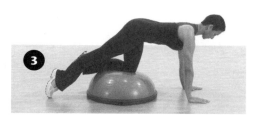

1 Extend and lift your right leg so that it's parallel to the floor.

2 Extend and lift your left arm straight in front of you. Keep your head in line with your spine. Hold for 2 counts.

3 Lower your arm and leg to their starting positions.

Repeat 4–5 times, then start over on the other side.

BASIC
Keep the toes of your back foot down to help you balance.

CHALLENGE
As you extend and lift your opposite arm and leg, bend the extended arm and draw your elbow and knee as close as possible in toward your chest, rounding your back at the same time.

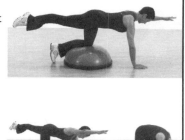

TIPS

- Make sure your hands are under your shoulders and your knees are under your hips.
- Keep your head in line with your spine.
- Focus on a spot on the floor in front of you.

STARTING POSITION: Stand on the dome with your left foot on the bull's eye and your right foot touching the side of the dome. Raise your arms out to the sides in a T.

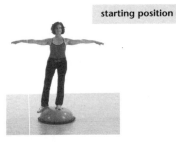

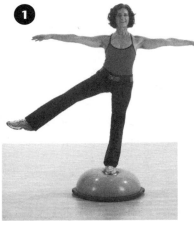

1 Keep your upper body still as you extend and lift your right leg to the side. Focus on a point straight ahead to help you balance. Hold for 2 counts.

2 Lower your leg to its starting position.

Repeat 4–5 times, then start over on the other side.

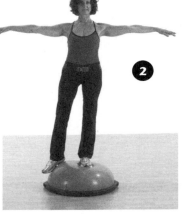

BASIC

Rest your leg on the outside rim of the dome and slide it from the front around to the back. Also try practicing on the floor before trying the exercise on the BOSU.

TIPS

• Engage your inner thigh muscles to help you stand firmly on your supporting leg.

STARTING POSITION: Sit with your hips and buttocks toward the back of the platform. Bend your knees and place your feet flat on the floor in front of you.

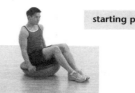

starting position

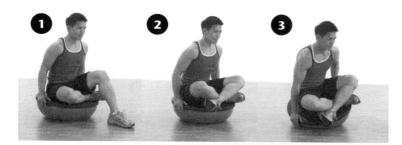

1 Hold the side handles and slowly lift your right leg to the platform. Carefully bend your knee and rest the side of your right calf on the surface.

2 Slowly lift and fold your left leg to the platform. Adjust your position so that you are balanced and sitting cross-legged.

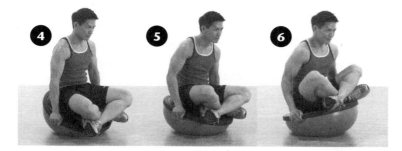

3 Without changing your position, engage your core and shift your weight toward the right to tilt the BOSU to the right.

4 Stay connected to your core and shift your weight toward the front to tilt the BOSU forward.

BASIC

Do the exercise while sitting on top of the platform with your knees bent and your feet on the floor.

CHALLENGE

Smooth out the hip tilts to a continuous hip circle to the left and then to the right.

SUPER CHALLENGE

Try the hip circles with your arms in a T.

5 Stay connected and shift your weight toward the left to tilt the BOSU to the left.

6 Stay connected and shift your weight toward the back to tilt the BOSU backward.

Repeat steps 3–6 several times.

TIPS

• Keep your spine long and your shoulders over your hips.

STARTING POSITION: Sit with your hips and buttocks toward the back of the platform. Bend your knees and place your feet flat on the floor in front of you.

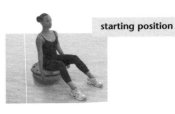

starting position

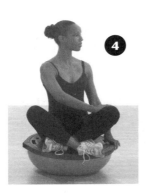

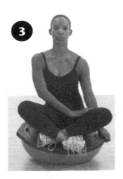

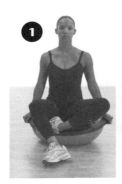

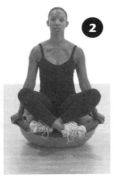

1 Hold the side handles and slowly lift your left leg to the platform. Carefully bend your knee and rest the side of your left calf on the surface.

2 Slowly lift and fold your right leg to the platform. Adjust your position so that you are balanced and sitting cross-legged.

3 Place your right hand on top of your left thigh.

4 Lift out of your hips and twist toward your left.

5 Place your left hand behind you on the platform surface or rim of the BOSU. Hold for 5 counts.

Start over on the other side.

Repeat 1–2 more times.

BASIC

Do the exercise with one leg folded underneath you on the platform and the other foot on the floor in front of you. Twist to one side and then the other.

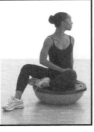

TIPS

• Keep your spine long and your head in line with your spine.

STARTING POSITION: Stand on the dome, centering your weight over your feet. Rest your hands by your sides and look straight ahead.

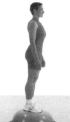

starting position

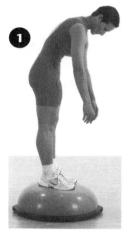

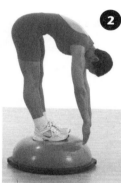

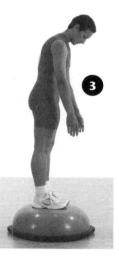

1 Engage your abs. At the same time, gently nod your chin to your chest to begin rolling sequentially toward your feet.

2 Continue rolling down. Go as far as you can while maintaining your balance and staying in your curl. Hold for 5 counts.

3 Slowly roll back to standing one vertebra at a time. Your head should come up last.

Repeat 4–5 times.

CHALLENGE

Twist to your right and roll down toward your right foot as if you're curling over a big beach ball with one arm forward and one arm back (like the Atlas statue). Keep both knees bent as you roll down and roll back up to standing.

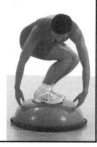

TIPS

- Keep your neck long and relaxed and your head in line with your spine.
- Engage your core vigorously and avoid buckling at the hips.
- For added stability, engage your inner thighs but keep your knees over your toes.

exercises with weights

The benefits of weight or resistance training are well documented. In addition to the obvious gains in muscular strength, using weights speeds up metabolism, burns calories faster, and helps prevent osteoporosis, a loss of bone density that increases the risk of fractures.

Using weights or weighted balls intensifies the effects of the BOSU, especially where balance and weight distribution are concerned. Weights force you to use offsetting and core muscles to a far greater extent than would otherwise be the case. For this reason, it's a good idea to start with light weights or balls—2 or 3 pounds are sufficient. Then progress to heavier ones if you wish. Good results are achievable even with fairly light weights, and you can always opt to do the exercises without weights if you prefer.

Helpful hints

- Only use as much weight as you can accommodate without straining or losing your form.
- Connect to your core and brace yourself at all times.
- Keep your shoulders away from your ears and your head in line with your spine.
- Keep your spine in neutral and avoid arching your lower back.
- Avoid ballistic or jerky movements.
- Don't hold your breath! Exhale during the exertion.

STARTING POSITION: Stand on the dome with your feet about hip-width apart and your knees slightly bent. Hold a free weight in each hand at your sides.

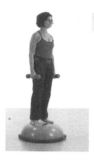

starting position

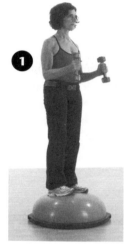

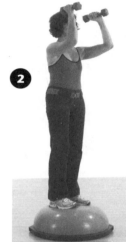

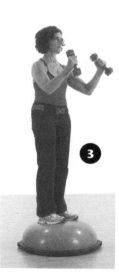

1 Hug your elbows in to your waist and lift your forearms so that they're parallel to the floor.

2 Without changing the shape of your arms, raise both arms up until your hands point to the ceiling and your upper arms are parallel to the floor. Hold for 2 counts.

3 Lower your arms back to their starting position.

Repeat 4–5 times.

CHALLENGE

Squat down at the same time as you raise your arms.

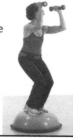

TIPS

- Engage your core, especially your abs, to stabilize.
- Keep your head in line with your spine and look straight ahead.
- Make sure your knees are over your toes, especially as you squat.

STARTING POSITION: Stand on the dome with your feet about hip-width apart and your arms by your sides. Hold a free weight in each hand.

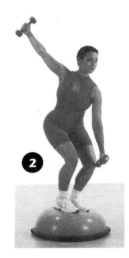

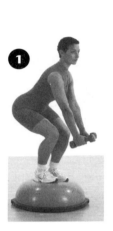

starting position

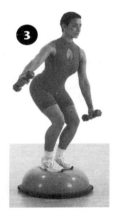

1 Squat down on the dome, going only as low as you can without rounding or arching your back. At the same time, extend both arms down toward your left hip (at about a 45° angle).

2 Without moving your hips, twist from your waist to the right. At the same time, open your right arm to the right (i.e., like opening a door). Hold for 2 counts.

3 Twist back to center and lower your arm.

Repeat steps 2–3 (the twist) 4–5 times, then start over on the other side.

CHALLENGE

Try the same exercise from a lunge position, keeping your back leg bent. For extra support, rest the elbow of your left arm on your left knee when you rotate to the right and vice versa.

SUPER CHALLENGE

Follow the hand weight with your eyes as you twist.

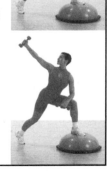

TIPS

• Engage your glutes, abs, and inner thighs to help keep your center of gravity as you twist.

STARTING POSITION: Kneel on top of the dome, centering your right knee on the bull's eye and extending your left leg straight behind you with your foot on the floor. Rest your left hand on the floor in front of the dome. Hold a free weight in your right hand.

starting position

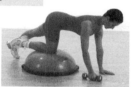

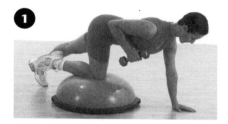

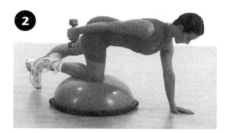

1 Bend your right elbow and lift the weight straight up. Stop when your fist is at your chest and your elbow is at your waist.

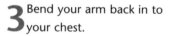

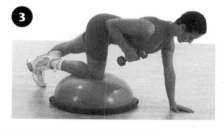

2 Straighten your right arm and press it back, keeping your elbow in line with your shoulder. Exhale to connect to your core as you press. Hold for 2 counts.

3 Bend your arm back in to your chest.

Repeat 5–10 times, then start over on the other side.

BASIC
Do the exercise with both knees on top of the dome.

CHALLENGE
Lift the leg that's extended to the back up to hip height. Repeat the exercise in this position.

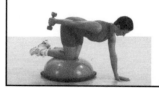

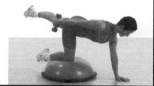

TIPS
- Keep your spine long from head to tailbone.
- Avoid looking down or dropping your chin to your chest.

kneeling short-lever fly

STARTING POSITION: Kneel upright on top of the dome with your knees on either side of the bull's eye and your toes off the floor. Hold a free weight in each hand at your sides.

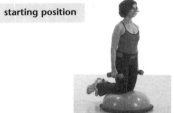

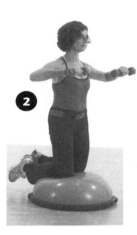

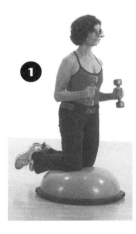

1 Hug your elbows in to your waist and lift your forearms so that they're parallel to the floor.

2 Without changing the shape of your arms, arc your elbows out to the sides until your upper arms are in line with your shoulders. Hold for 2 counts.

3 Lower your arms back down and hug your elbows in to your waist again.

Repeat 5–10 times.

BASIC
Do the exercise with your toes down to help you balance.

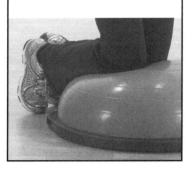

TIPS
- Engage your abs to protect your back and help you balance.
- Keep your back straight and strong. Reach the crown of your head toward the ceiling.

Caution: Avoid this exercise if you have shoulder or wrist problems.

STARTING POSITION: Place your right knee on the bull's eye and extend your left leg straight back with your toes on the floor. Hold a free weight in each hand and rest them on a mat or other non-slip surface in front of the dome. Keep your arms straight and directly under your shoulders.

starting position
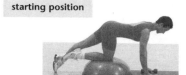

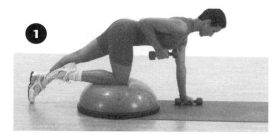

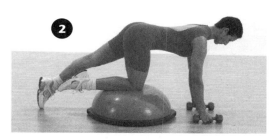

1 Bend your right elbow and lift your right hand and weight straight up until your fist reaches your chest. Hold for 2 counts.

2 Lower the arm back to its starting position.

Repeat 5–10 times, then start over on the other side.

BASIC

Keep your toes down to help you balance. It may also help to practice on the floor first.

CHALLENGE

Lift your extended leg to hip height and repeat the exercise in this position.

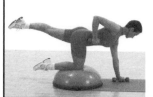

SUPER CHALLENGE

Instead of doing a one-arm row, extend your active arm straight out in front of you at shoulder height and hold for 2 counts. Then arc it out to the side and hold for 2 counts.

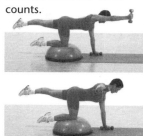

TIPS

- Press your hands into the weights to avoid sinking between your shoulder blades.
- Engage your abs to protect your back and help you balance.
- Keep your back straight and strong. Keep your head in line with your spine.

kneeling lateral arm raise

STARTING POSITION: Kneel upright on top of the dome with your knees on either side of the bull's eye and your toes off the floor behind you. Hold a free weight in each hand at your sides.

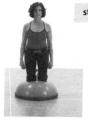

starting position

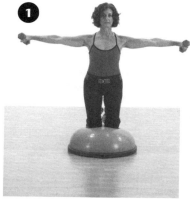

1

1 Keep your neck long and shoulders down as you lift your arms to a T. Hold for 2 counts.

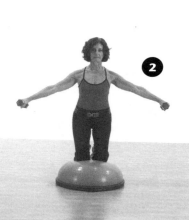

2

2 Lower your arms back to their starting position.

Repeat 5–10 times.

BASIC
Keep your toes down to help you balance.

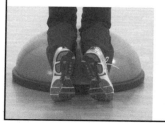

SUPER CHALLENGE
Bend and lift one knee to the side and repeat the exercise in this position. Make sure your supporting knee is on the bull's eye. Engage your core like crazy!

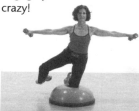

TIPS
- Draw your inner thighs together to help you stabilize.
- Engage your abs to protect your back and avoid buckling at your hips.
- Keep your back straight and your head in line with your spine.

fly in bridge

STARTING POSITION: Assume a bridge position: Your upper back, shoulders, and head rest on the platform; your hips are lifted, knees are bent, and feet are flat on the floor; weight is evenly distributed between your feet and across your shoulders. Hold a free weight in each hand and extend your arms over your chest, pointing your fists to the ceiling.

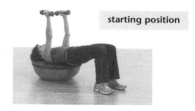
starting position

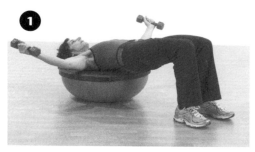

1 Press your shoulders into the platform and use your chest muscles to open your arms to the sides. Keep your elbows soft and do not go below shoulder height. Hold for 2 counts.

2 Lift your arms back up over your chest. Hold for 2 counts.

Repeat 5–10 times.

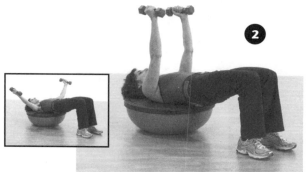

CHALLENGE
Try a one-arm fly, starting with your right arm. Be sure to brace yourself, or you'll roll to the side. Repeat on the other side.

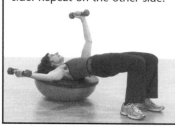

TIPS
• Keep your abs tight and use your glutes and hamstrings to keep your hips up.

close-grip triceps press in bridge

STARTING POSITION: Assume a bridge position: Your upper back, shoulders, and head rest on the platform; your hips are lifted, knees are bent, and feet are flat on the floor; weight is evenly distributed between your feet and across your shoulders. Hold a free weight in each hand at your sides.

starting position

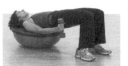

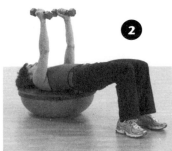

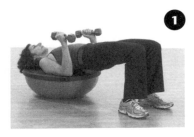

1 Hug your elbows in to your sides. At the same time, bend your elbows until your fists point to the ceiling and the backs of your upper arms rest on the platform beside your torso.

2 Exhale and, using resistance, push your arms up to the ceiling until they're straight. Keep your elbows close to your body and avoid locking them.

3 Using resistance, lower your upper arms back down beside your torso.

Repeat steps 2–3 several times.

TIPS
- Keep your abs tight.
- Use your glutes and hamstrings to keep your hips up.

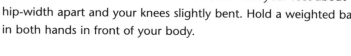

STARTING POSITION: Stand on the dome with your feet about hip-width apart and your knees slightly bent. Hold a weighted ball in both hands in front of your body.

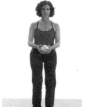

starting position

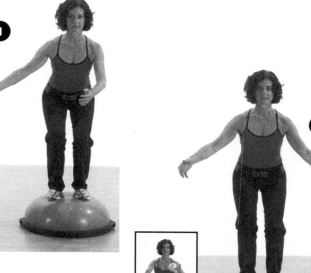

1 Bend down into a squat position and transfer the weighted ball to your right hand.

2 Pass the weighted ball back to your left hand in front of your torso. Then continue to pass the ball back and forth from one hand to the other.

Repeat several times.

BASIC

Do the exercise with a small unweighted ball first.

CHALLENGE

Try following the ball back and forth with your eyes as you pass it from one hand to the other.

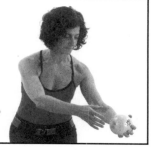

TIPS

- Engage your core and avoid buckling at the hips.
- Only work with a weight that you can control.

STARTING POSITION: Stand on the dome with your feet about hip-width apart and your knees slightly bent. Hold a weighted ball in both hands in front of your body.

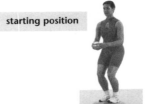

starting position

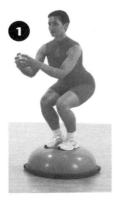

1

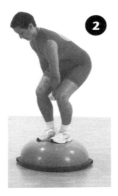

2

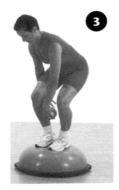

3

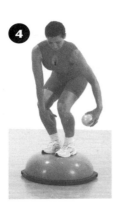

4

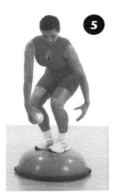

5

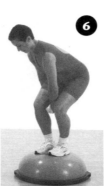

6

1 Bend down into a squat position.

2 Trace a figure-8 pattern through your legs. Start by holding the ball in your right hand behind your right knee.

3 Hold your left hand in front of your left leg and pass the ball to your left hand between your knees.

4 Pass the ball around the outside of your left leg to behind your left knee.

5 Hold your right hand in front of your right leg and pass the ball to your right hand between your knees.

6 Pass the ball around the outside of your right leg to behind your right knee to return to your starting position.

Repeat 4–5 times, then start over on the other side.

BASIC
Do the exercise with a small unweighted ball first.

CHALLENGE
Stay in your squat and start tracing your figure 8 at your knees, then move down to your calves, then down to your ankles, and back up again.

TIPS
- Engage your core vigorously to keep your body from rotating from side to side.
- Make sure your knees are above your toes.

STARTING POSITION: Sit with your hips centered on top of the dome. Place your feet about hip-width apart and flat on the floor. Leaning your torso back slightly, hold a weighted ball in both hands in front of your body.

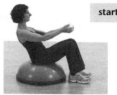

starting position

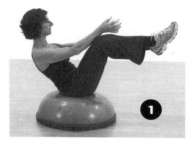

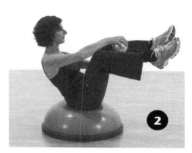

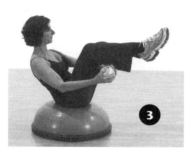

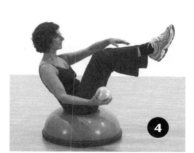

1 Engage your lower abs vigorously and lean back slightly. Then bend and lift your legs so that your shins are parallel to the floor.

2 Trace a figure-8 pattern through your legs. Start by holding the ball in your right hand by your right knee and your left hand in front of your left leg. Pass the ball between your knees to your left hand.

3 With your left hand, pass the ball around the outside of your left leg to behind your left knee, then pass the ball between your knees to your right hand.

4 With your right hand, pass the ball around the outside of your right leg to behind your right knee to return to the start of the figure 8.

Repeat 4–5 times, then start over on the other side.

BASIC

Do the exercise with a small unweighted ball first. Also try holding the ball in front with both feet on the floor or do the sequence with one leg up at a time.

CHALLENGE

Challenge your balance and move your leg up as you pass the ball under it and down as you pass the ball over it.

TIPS

- Engage your core vigorously to keep your body from rotating from side to side.

stretches

Muscles contract when they work. Stretching lengthens contracted muscle tissue and increases the flow of blood to remove waste and provide nutrients. Stretching also improves flexibility by increasing the range of motion in our joints. Stretching helps us stay mobile and reduces the risk of injury, especially as we age.

Keep in mind that it's possible to overstretch. You should therefore stretch only until you feel a certain amount of tension or a slight pulling, but no pain. Ideally it's a good idea to stretch all major muscle groups slowly and with control, holding each stretch for 20 to 30 seconds.

Helpful hints

- Stretch your muscles when they're warm—after a workout or at least 5 minutes of cardiovascular exercise.
- Always ease into a stretch. Never bounce, force, or overstretch. Your body will tell you how far to go.
- Breathing, especially exhaling, helps muscles release. Take slow, deep breaths in through your nose and out through your mouth.
- Take your time to set up properly. Alignment is key in any stretching position.
- Drink lots of water. Proper hydration enhances flexibility and helps relax the body.

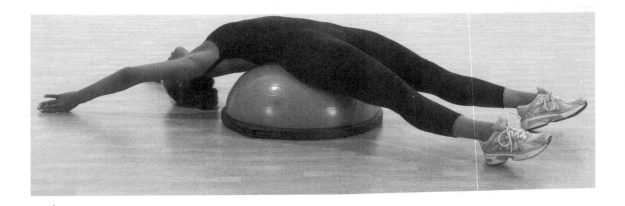

STARTING POSITION: Kneel with your left knee centered on top of the dome. Bend your right knee and place your right foot on the floor in front of the dome.

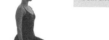

starting position

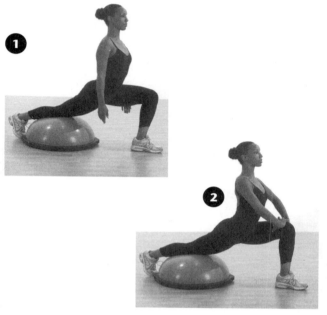

1 Walk your right leg farther out to the front and bend your knee at right angles, making sure your right knee is over your ankle. Lean forward enough to feel a stretch in the front of your left hip.

2 Place your hands on your right thigh and press down slightly to add resistance and lengthen your spine. Hold for a minimum of 20 seconds.

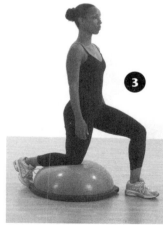

3 Return to your starting position.

Start over on the other side.

BASIC
For added support, use a prop, such as a body bar, broomstick, or the wall.

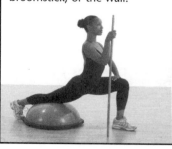

STARTING POSITION: Stand a comfortable distance behind the dome with your feet about hip-width apart. Rest your hands by your sides.

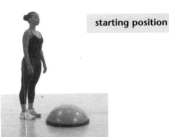
starting position

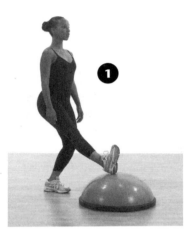

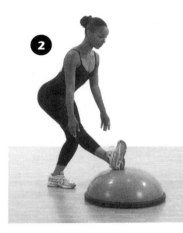

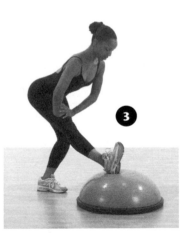

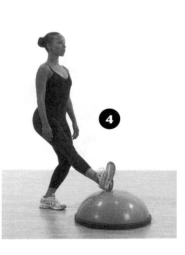

1 Bend your left knee. At the same time, extend your right leg and place your right heel on top of the dome. Flex your foot and make sure your right leg is straight.

2 With a straight back, hinge forward from your hips to stretch your right hamstring and calf muscles.

3 Place your hands on your right thigh and press down slightly to add resistance and lengthen your spine. Hold for a minimum of 20 seconds.

4 Straighten up and return to your starting position.

Start over on the other side.

TIPS
• Keep your head in line with your spine.

STARTING POSITION: Stand a comfortable distance behind the dome with your feet about hip-width apart. Rest your hands by your sides.

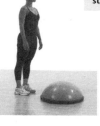

starting position

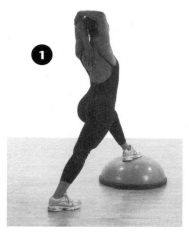

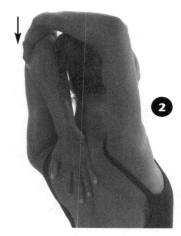

1 Assume a lunge position with your left foot on the dome, and hold your left elbow so that it points to the ceiling above your left shoulder.

2 Point the fingers of your left hand down your back toward the floor and gently press your left elbow toward your left hand. Hold for a minimum of 20 seconds.

3 Release your hands and return to your starting position.

Start over on the other side.

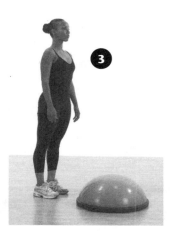

BASIC
Do the stretch while kneeling on the dome instead of from a lunge.

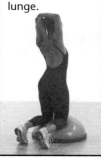

TIPS
• Avoid arching your back and popping your ribs forward.

stretches
back release

STARTING POSITION: Sit with your hips centered on top of the dome. Bend your knees and place your feet flat on the floor in front of you.

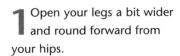

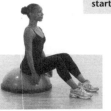

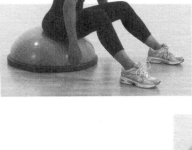

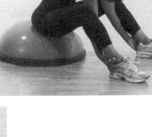

1 Open your legs a bit wider and round forward from your hips.

2 Bend your arms and bring them to the insides of your legs. Wrap your hands around the outsides of your ankles and rest your hands on the tops of your feet.

3 Let your head hang to release your neck and upper back. Hold for a minimum of 20 seconds.

4 Roll up to your starting position.

Repeat if desired.

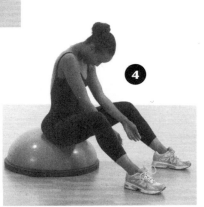

TIPS
- Gently press your upper arms into your knees and contract your lower abs to open your lower back and increase the stretch.

Caution: Avoid this stretch if you have ankle or knee problems.

STARTING POSITION: Kneel behind the BOSU, facing it.

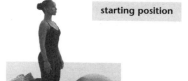

starting position

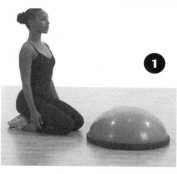

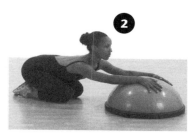

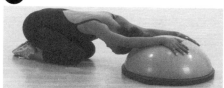

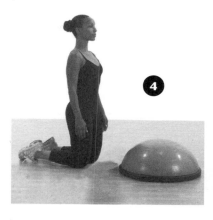

1 Sit back on your heels.

2 Extend your arms in front of you and place your hands on top of the dome.

3 Lower your head and rest it on the dome or let it hang to release your neck and upper back. Hold for a minimum of 20 seconds.

4 Roll up to your starting position.

Repeat if desired.

CHALLENGE
Try the same exercise with your arms extended diagonally to the side to stretch the oblique muscles on your sides.

STARTING POSITION: Sit with your hips toward the front edge of the dome. Bend your knees and place your feet flat on the floor in front of you. Rest your hands by your sides.

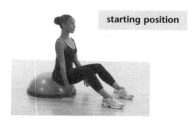

starting position

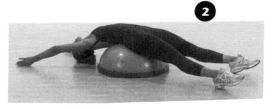

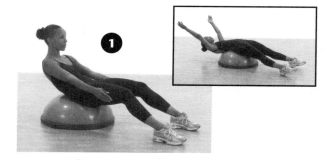

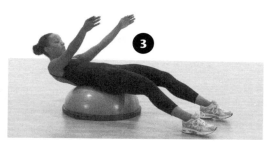

1 Slowly roll back and extend your upper body over the dome. At the same time, arc your arms back to a V behind you and let your head hang toward the floor.

2 Straighten your legs in front of you. Hold for a minimum of 20 seconds.

3 Roll up to your starting position.

Repeat if desired.

BASIC

Sit on the floor in front of the dome and lie back as far as you can. If desired, add a pillow under your head for more support. Extend your arms to the sides instead of to a V.

STARTING POSITION: Sit with your hips centered on top of the dome and your legs open to a straddle position. Go as far as you can without bending your knees and rounding your lower back.

starting position

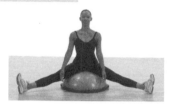

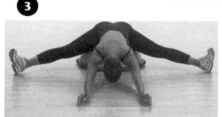

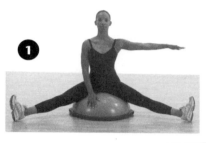

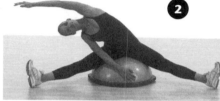

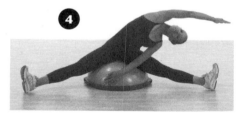

1 Place your right hand on the dome between your legs and lift your left arm out to the side.

2 Do a side bend toward your right: Extend your left hand over your head, reaching toward where the wall and ceiling meet. Hold for a minimum of 20 seconds then straighten up to center.

3 Hinge forward from your hips and stretch out in front. Keep your back flat and reach straight ahead with your arms. Hold for a minimum of 20 seconds then straighten up to center.

4 Do a side bend to your left: Extend your right hand over your head. Hold for a minimum of 20 seconds then straighten up to center.

Repeat if desired.

TIPS

- Avoid collapsing and rounding your lower back.
- Keep your spine straight and lift out of your hips as you stretch.

part 4:
the
workouts

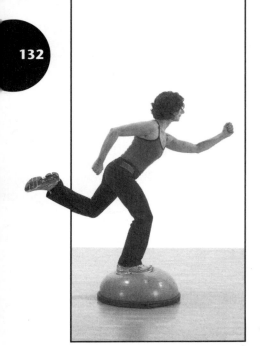

ready for blast-off

The following workouts are based on exercises presented throughout the book. There are three targeted workouts (Core Blast, Lower Body Blast, and Torso Blast) as well as two complete workouts, both with a warm-up, a full-body workout consisting of selected exercises from each section of Part 3, and a cool-down with stretches.

Each workout shows a thumbnail of the exercise together with the page number where it appears in the book. In most cases, the thumbnails show the main version of the exercise. Feel free to substitute one of the other variations if you prefer.

Before you start

Before you attempt any of the workouts that follow, warm up your body with 5 to 10 minutes of low-impact cardio exercises using a treadmill, exercise bike, or elliptical machine if possible. Otherwise, follow the warm-ups in the Complete Workouts later in this section.

core blast

The Core Blast focuses mainly on the abs and core, using exercises from the Abs and Core section as well as the side exercises in the Plank, Push-up, and Side section.

CORE BLAST

lower body blast

The Lower Body Blast workout combines exercises from the Squats and Lunges section and the kneeling exercises in the Kneeling and Balance section.

LOWER BODY BLAST

	PAGE	EXERCISE
	58	squat and over-the-top combo
	60	squat and twist combo
	62	side-squat combo
	63	squat and leg-lift combo
	64	squat and jump combo
	65	kickboxing squat combo
	102	knee lift
	103	kneeling crunch
	104	kneeling tracking drill
	105	kneeling with leg and arm extension
	66	backward lunge
	67	side lunge
	68	forward lunge
	69	lunge forward and back

torso blast

The Torso Blast contains exercises from the Back and Bridge section as well as the Plank, Push-up, and Side Exercises section.

TORSO BLAST

	PAGE	EXERCISE
	88	platform hip roll from bridge
	89	one-legged balance in bridge
	90	ab curl in shoulder bridge
	83	swimming
	84	airplane balance
	85	spinal extension with twist
	86	swan dive
	87	leg push
	92	dome plank
	93	platform plank
	94	lunge from plank
	95	dome push-up
	96	platform push-up

complete workout 1

Complete Workout 1 is designed to engage your whole body. It starts with a warm-up consisting of exercises from Part 2 BOSU Basics and then presents selected exercises from each section of Part 3, ending with some stretches for a cool-down. Allow at least 45 minutes to an hour for this workout, depending on the speed of your reps and the length of your rest periods.

COMPLETE WORKOUT 1

warm-ups

PAGE	EXERCISE
28	standing on the dome
28	standing on the dome—eyes closed (challenge)
37	side tap to side lunge
26	stepping up and down—slow and faster (basic)
26	stepping up and down—arm swings (challenge)
27	basic knee lift
38	stepping on the dome
38	marching on the dome (challenge)
38	jogging on the dome (super challenge)
36	squatting on the dome
36	squatting on the dome—arm circles (challenge)

cardio

PAGE	EXERCISE
53	two-foot jump
53	two-foot jump—random (super challenge)
45	power knee
46	3 knee repeater
52	knee to chest

COMPLETE WORKOUT 1 *continued*

tone & balance

	PAGE	EXERCISE
	62	side-squat combo
	64	squat and jump combo
	54	turning jumps
	56	mogul jumps
	66	backward lunge
	67	side lunge
	119	weighted ball pass
	120	standing figure 8
	111	arm curl
	112	golf swing squat
	106	single-leg balance
	109	roll down
	114	kneeling short-lever fly
	116	kneeling lateral arm raise
	102	knee lift
	104	kneeling tracking drill
	98	side curl
	99	lateral leg lift
	83	swimming
	85	spinal extension with twist

COMPLETE WORKOUT 1 *continued*

	PAGE	EXERCISE
	88	platform hip roll from bridge
	93	platform plank
	94	lunge from plank
	96	platform push-up
	90	ab curl in shoulder bridge
	74	curl and leg-extension combo
	78	double-leg stretch
	79	supine lean
	81	pike up
	124	hamstring and calf stretch
	126	back release
	129	side stretch

stretches

complete workout 2

Like Complete Workout 1, Complete Workout 2 is also designed to engage your whole body. It starts with a warm-up consisting of different exercises from Part 2 BOSU Basics, but this time the warm-up starts on the knees. After the warm-up is a different selection of exercises from each section of Part 3, ending with a few stretches for a cool-down. Allow at least 45 minutes to an hour for this workout, depending on the speed of your reps and the length of your rest periods.

COMPLETE WORKOUT 2

warm-ups

	PAGE	EXERCISE
	30	kneeling tall
	31	kneeling on all fours
	34	single-leg extension
	34	single-leg extension—opposite arm/leg (challenge)
	35	simple back extension
	32	pelvic tilt
	33	hip roll in bridge
	28	standing on the dome
	28	standing on the dome—closed eyes (challenge)
	29	side twist
	29	side twist—weighted ball (super challenge)
	39	single-foot forward jump
	40	single-foot sideways jump
	26	stepping up and down—slow and faster (basic)
	26	stepping up and down—arm swings (challenge)

	PAGE	EXERCISE
cardio	48	L-step/leg-curl combo
	50	front leg kick
	51	side leg kick
	60	squat and twist combo
	63	squat and leg-lift combo
	57	tuck jump
	55	cross-country switch jumps
	58	squat and over-the-top combo
	65	kickboxing squat combo
	68	forward lunge
	68	forward lunge—exchange (super challenge)
	69	lunge forward and back
tone & balance	71	ab curl
	90	ab curl in shoulder bridge
	72	leg exchange
	73	criss-cross
	80	supine extension
	89	one-legged balance in bridge
	117	fly in bridge
	118	close-grip triceps press in bridge

	PAGE	EXERCISE
	75	v-sit series
	121	v-sit figure 8
	76	bent-leg rotation
	77	seated leg exchange
	97	side balance
	100	side lift
	84	airplane balance
	86	swan dive
	87	leg push
	107	hip circles
	108	seated spinal twist
	103	kneeling crunch
	105	kneeling with leg and arm extension
	113	kneeling triceps press
	115	kneeling one-arm row
	92	dome plank
	95	dome push-up
	123	hip flexor stretch
	125	triceps stretch
	127	back stretch: child's pose
	128	back extension

stretches

resources

Books

Abs on the Ball. Rochester, VT: Healing Arts Press, 2003.

Blahnik, Jay, and Douglas Brooks and Candice Copeland Brooks. *BOSU Balance Trainer Complete Workout System*. BOSU Fitness LLC, 2006.

Brooks, Douglas, M.S. and Candice Copeland Brooks. *BOSU Balance Trainer Integrated Balance Training*. DW Fitness LLC, 2002.

Craig, Colleen. *Pilates on the Ball*. Rochester, VT: Healing Arts Press, 2001.

Elphinston, Joanne, and Paul Pook. *The Core Workout*. Core Workout, 1999.

Jemmett, Rick. *The Athlete's Ball*. Halifax: Novont Health Publishing, 2004.

Marinovich, Marv and Edythe M. Heus. *ProBodX*. New York: HarperCollins, 2003.

McGill, Stuart. *Ultimate Back Fitness and Performance*. Waterloo: Backfitpro Inc., 2006.

Nelson, Miriam, and Sarah Wernick. *Strong Women, Strong Bones*. New York: Perigree, 2000.

Posner-Mayer, Joanne. *Swiss Ball Applications for Orthopedic and Sports Medicine*. Longmont, CO: Ball Dynamics International, 1995.

Potvin, Andre Noel, and Chad Benson. *The Great Balance & Stability Handbook*. Surrey, BC: Productive Fitness Products Inc., 2003.

Strength Training on the Ball. Rochester, VT: Healing Arts Press, 2005.

Richardson, Carolyn, Gwendolyn Jull, Julie Hides, and Paul Hodges. *Therapeutic Exercise for Spinal Segmental Stabilization in Low Back Pain*. London: Churchill Livingstone, 1999.

Ungaro, Alycea. *Pilates Body in Motion*. New York: DK Publishing, 2002.

Websites

www.bosufitness.com

www.bosu.com

www.mayoclinic.com/health/core-exercises/ SM00071

DVDs

Blahnik, Jay. *BOSU Equilibrium*. DW Fitness LLC, 2003.

Brooks, Douglas. *BOSU Strength and Athletic Conditioning for Personal Trainers*. DW Fitness LLC, 2003.

Brooks, Douglas, and Jennifer Cole, Candice Brooks and David Weck. *BOSU Balance Trainer Total Body Workout*. BOSU Fitness LLC, 2004 and 2006.

Copeland Brooks, Candice. *BOSU Core Synergy*. DW Fitness LLC, 2003.

Gaspar, Gay. *BOSU Reactive Strength and Power*. DW Fitness LLC, 2003.

Glick, Rob. *BOSU CardioFusion*. DW Fitness LLC, 2003.

Mylrea, Mindy. *BOSU Total Sports Conditioning*. DW Fitness LLC, 2003.

index

about the authors

COLLEEN CRAIG, a certified Pilates trainer and ballet dancer, studied the Pilates Method with Moira Stott at the Stott International Training and Certification Centre in Canada. Her books include *Pilates on the Ball: A Comprehensive Book and DVD Workout* and *Strength Training on the Ball: A Pilates Approach to Optimal Strength and Balance*. She lives in Toronto.

MIRIANE TAYLOR has been a certified Pilates instructor and teacher trainer for the past 20 years. She was one of the original teachers at the well-known Stott Pilates Studios in Toronto. A former dancer and choreographer, Miriane now runs her own Pilates and training studio in Toronto (www.taylor-dpilates.com) and teaches workshops both at home and internationally.

JANE ARONOVITCH is a BOSU® enthusiast as well as a certified Gyrokinesis® instructor, a Pilates, yoga, and Gyrotonic® practitioner, and a former folkdance teacher, choreographer, and performer. She also runs a successful business producing all kinds of business, technical, and training materials (www.seejanewrite.com).

about the photographer

ANDY MOGG is a well-known and much-published photographer. Born in England in 1954, he worked as a consultant, then writer and photographer. At 17, he moved from London to Belgium, traveling and working his way through Europe; he settled in the United States 20 years ago. He now runs a thriving photography studio in Oakland, California. For more information, visit his website at www.dancingimages.com.